Menopause Diet

Discover the Power of Nutrition and Herbal Remedies to Boost Metabolism, Improve Mood, and Love Your Body

By

Lesley Loss

Table of Contents

The information herein is offered for informational purposes solely and is universal as so. The presentation of the information is without a contract or any type of guarantee assurance.

The trademarks that are used are without any consent, and the publication of the trademark is without permission or backing by the trademark owner. All trademarks and brands within this book are for clarifying purposes only and are owned by the owners themselves, not affiliated with this document.

Table of Contents

About the Author

My name is Lesley and I have a passion for healthy living and holistic practices. I strive every day to improve my life and the lives of my loved ones through actions that I believe are good for the body and mind.

I am also interested in healthy diets, nutrition and gardening. In particular, I love growing organic foods. I have found that they fit perfectly with my lifestyle, which I try to keep as healthy as possible.

I grew up in a large family, and although we didn't have a lot of money we always managed to bring healthy and natural foods to our table. These habits are what led me to try to convey my food values to a wider audience than just my immediate family.

Another key part of my life is physical activity, which I consider to be of extraordinary importance for my health. Maybe it's because I have always been accustomed to long runs or walks throughout my childhood, hikes that I used to take while walking up and down the fields that surrounded my home.

Now I am a mom of two wonderful children, to whom I am trying to instill the culture of healthy eating, but without too much pressure. I love it all and I love this life. I hope with all my heart to pass it on to all of you as well through the pages of these books of mine.

Introduction

This book is designed to be your trusted companion as you navigate the transformative journey of menopause, providing you with valuable insights, practical strategies, and delicious recipes to optimize your health and well-being during this unique phase of life.

Transition in a woman's life, marking the end of her reproductive years. It is a normal and inevitable process that occurs as a woman reaches a certain stage of maturity. It brings about significant changes in hormonal balance, it also opens up new opportunities for self-care, personal growth, and vibrant health. Understanding how your body responds to these changes and nourishing it with the right foods can make all the difference in alleviating symptoms, enhancing your overall well-being, and empowering you to live peacefully during this period.

In this book, we will explore foods' powerful impact on menopause symptoms and how you can make informed dietary choices to support your body's needs.

You'll discover which foods to embrace and which to avoid as we delve into the science behind their effects on hormonal balance, mood swings, hot flashes, weight management, and more.

While nutrition forms the foundation of the Menopause Diet, we'll also delve into other essential aspects of holistic wellness. Menopause is a time of immense physical and emotional change, and it's crucial to approach it with self-compassion, understanding, and mindfulness. Throughout this book, you will find practical guidance on how to live peacefully during this transformative period, cultivating self-care practices, managing stress, and embracing the journey with grace.

To make your menopause journey even more enjoyable, we have included a collection of delicious and nourishing recipes. These recipes are thoughtfully crafted to incorporate the right foods, herbs, and natural remedies to relieve symptoms and support your overall well-being. From hormone-balancing smoothies to satisfying main dishes and delightful snacks, these recipes will inspire you to nourish yourself with love and care. Additionally, we will explore the physiological processes that occur during menopause, empowering you with knowledge and understanding.

By demystifying the intricacies of menopause, we aim to equip you with the tools to make informed decisions about your health and confidently embrace this transition.

It's important to note that this book is not about quick fixes or miraculous cures. Instead, it is a comprehensive guide that encourages you to adopt sustainable lifestyle changes and harness the power of natural remedies to support your well-being. By embracing the Menopause Diet, you will learn how to avoid weight gain caused by hormonal changes and achieve a healthy body through proper nutrition and mindful living.

Whether you are just entering perimenopause or have already embraced the full spectrum of menopausal changes, this book empowers you. It will be a trusted companion, providing you with the knowledge, tools, and inspiration you need to thrive during this remarkable chapter of your life.

Together, let us embark on this transformative journey, nourishing our bodies, minds, and spirits with love, understanding, and the power of the Menopause Diet.

Chapter 1: What Is Menopause and it's Stages?

Menopause, a biologically normal process, signals the conclusion of a woman's fertile years. It is described as the complete cessation of menstruation for 12 straight months due to the ovaries producing fewer hormones. With an average age of 51, menopause typically hits around 45 and 55.

Perimenopause refers to the phases before menopause as a whole. Perimenopause may start years before menopause, distinguished by erratic menstrual cycles and shifting hormone levels. Women may have various symptoms during this phase, including vaginal dryness, night sweats, hot flashes, mood swings, disturbed sleep, and decreased libido.

1.1 Menopause Stages

The real phases of menopause may be divided into the following categories:

- Pre-menopause refers to the stage preceding perimenopause when a woman normally ovulates and has regular menstrual cycles. Menopause is still some years away, and hormone levels remain rather constant.

- The time preceding menopause is known as perimenopause. During this time, hormone levels, notably those of estrogen and progesterone, vary more noticeably, causing irregular periods and the start of several menopausal symptoms.

- Menopause: After a year without a monthly cycle, menopause is formally identified. The amount of progesterone and estrogen produced by the ovaries has drastically decreased. During this phase, menopausal symptoms may persist and extend for years.

- After menopause, a woman has post-menopause for the remainder of her life. It describes the years that come after menopause when the body has had time to acclimate to hormone alterations. While some women may endure long-term consequences, including vaginal dryness, a decline in bone density, and a higher likelihood of certain medical diseases, menopausal symptoms generally fade.

It is essential to remember that each woman's menopausal experience is different. From person to person, symptoms may range widely in length and severity. While some women could find it relatively easy to go through these phases, others might find it more difficult. During this transforming period, seeking medical advice and assistance may help control symptoms and preserve general health.

1.2 What Causes Menopause to Happen?

As the ovaries age and produce fewer reproductive hormones, a natural process known as menopause occurs. Diminished levels of progesterone, estrogen, luteinizing hormone (LH), follicle-stimulating hormone (FSH), and testosterone, lead to significant changes in the body. One noticeable change is the absence of functioning ovarian follicles, which are responsible for the release of eggs and support menstruation and fertility.

For many women, the first sign of menopause is a decrease in the regularity of their menstrual periods, often accompanied by heavier and longer flows. This typically occurs in the late 40s or early 50s, with the average age of menopause being around 52 in American women. Menopause can also be induced by ovarian injury or surgical removal of the ovaries and surrounding pelvic tissues.

Induced menopause may occur due to bilateral oophorectomy, a surgical procedure that involves removing both ovaries. In some cases, ovarian function is deliberately suppressed in women with estrogen receptor-expressing malignancies through hormone therapy, surgery, radiation therapy, pelvic radiation, or procedures that damage or remove the ovaries.

1.3 How Is Menopause Identified?

If you have bothersome or incapacitating menopausal symptoms or signs of menopause and are forty-five years of age or younger, it is important to speak with your healthcare professional. The FDA and its Trusted Source just authorized a new blood test called the PicoAMH Elisa test for diagnosis. This examination evaluates if a woman has reached menopause or is on the verge of doing so.

Women who exhibit perimenopause symptoms, potentially harming health, may find this new test useful. An increased risk of osteoporosis, fractures, heart disease, cognitive decline, vaginal changes, libido loss, and mood swings is linked to early menopause.

A blood test that measures the blood levels of certain hormones, often FSH and an estrogen variant called estradiol, may also be prescribed by your doctor.

Menopause is often confirmed by persistently raised FSH levels in the blood of 30 mIU/mL or above and the absence of menstruation for a continuous year. Although they are both costly and inaccurate, saliva and OTC (over-the-counter) tests for urine are also available. Because FSH and estrogen levels change daily during perimenopause, most medical professionals will make a diagnosis based on the patient's symptoms, health history, and menstrual data. Your healthcare practitioner may also request further blood tests to help rule out any underlying disorders causing your symptoms based on the signs and medical history.

In addition, the following blood tests are often performed to confirm menopause:

- Tests for the function of the thyroid, blood lipid profile, the liver, the kidneys, and the thyroid.

- Tests for chorionic gonadotropin (HCG), estrogen, progesterone, prolactin, and progesterone

1.4 Home Remedies and Lifestyle Changes

Mild to moderate symptoms associated with menopause can be alleviated naturally through various methods, such as making lifestyle adjustments, trying home remedies, and exploring complementary therapies. Here are a few suggestions that you can implement at home to manage menopausal symptoms:

Regulating Body Temperature and Comfort

Opt for loose, layered clothing, especially at night and in warm or unpredictable weather, to help manage hot flashes.

Keep your bedroom cool, avoid heavy blankets, and consider using a waterproof sheet to protect your mattress if you experience night sweats.

Use a small fan to cool down when feeling overheated.

Maintaining Fitness and Managing Weight

Reduce daily calorie intake by 400 to 600 calories to help maintain weight.

Engage in 20 to 30 minutes of moderate physical activity each day to increase energy levels, promote better sleep, improve mood, and enhance overall well-being.

Addressing Emotional Needs

Seek support from a therapist or psychologist to discuss feelings of sadness, anxiety, depression, loneliness, insomnia, or identity changes.

Communicate your emotions of anxiety, mood swings, or sadness with your family, loved ones, or friends, so they can better understand and support you.

Enhancing Diet with Supplements

Consider taking magnesium, calcium, and vitamin D supplements to improve sleep quality, boost energy levels, and reduce the risk of osteoporosis. Consult your doctor for personalized recommendations.

Practicing Relaxation Techniques

Incorporate relaxation and breathing exercises like yoga, box breathing, and meditation into your routine.

Caring for Your Skin

Moisturize your skin daily to combat dryness, and avoid frequent bathing or swimming, as they can dry out or irritate the skin.

Addressing Sleep Problems

Temporarily use over-the-counter sleeping aids for insomnia or consult your doctor for natural sleep aids. Discuss persistent sleep issues with your doctor for further guidance.

Limiting Alcohol Consumption and Quitting Smoking

Quit smoking to avoid secondhand smoke, which can exacerbate symptoms.

Limit alcohol intake to prevent the worsening of symptoms and reduce the risk of developing health issues associated with heavy drinking during menopause.

Other Treatments

Some small studies have validated the use of herbal remedies to alleviate menopausal symptoms caused by estrogen deficiency.

Natural foods and supplements like soy, vitamin E, isoflavones, melatonin, and flaxseed may help reduce menopausal symptoms.

Black cohosh has been suggested to alleviate certain symptoms, but recent research evaluations have found limited evidence supporting these claims. Further studies are needed.

Claims that consuming omega-3 fatty acids can alleviate menopausal vasomotor symptoms lack solid evidence based on a reliable study conducted in 2015.

Chapter 2: Menopause Symptoms

Menopause, a biologically natural process, signifies the conclusion of a woman's reproductive years. During this transition, hormonal changes occur, leading to various symptoms that can impact daily life. The effects of these common menopausal symptoms on health and everyday activities are outlined below:

- Estrogen and progesterone changes:

o Night sweats and hot flashes: Excessive sweating and sudden sensations of heat can disrupt sleep, cause discomfort, and interfere with daily activities.

o Vaginal dryness and discomfort: Declining estrogen levels may result in dryness, itching, and pain during sexual activity, affecting intimate relationships.

o Changes in the menstrual cycle: Menstrual cycles during perimenopause may become irregular, heavier, or lighter, causing uncertainty and inconvenience.

- Physical and emotional symptoms:

o Mood swings, irritability, anxiety, and depression: Hormonal changes can contribute to emotional instability, making it challenging to regulate emotions and communicate effectively.

- Sleep disturbances:

o Night sweats, hot flashes, or mood swings can disrupt sleep, leading to decreased focus, daytime fatigue, and a reduced quality of life.

- Cognitive changes:

o Some women may experience memory lapses, trouble focusing, and "brain fog" during menopause, affecting daily functioning and work performance.

- Bone health and metabolism:

o Loss of bone density: The maintenance of bone density is heavily reliant on estrogen levels, and the decrease of estrogen during menopause raises the vulnerability to fractures and osteoporosis. Preserving bone health through nutrition, exercise, and possibly medication is essential.

o Weight gain and metabolic changes: Slowed metabolism during menopause can lead to weight gain, particularly in the waist and belly area, impacting self-esteem and body image.

- Heart health and general well-being:

o Higher risk of heart disease: Lower estrogen levels during menopause may elevate the risk of developing heart disease and other cardiovascular problems. Lifestyle changes and regular medical check-ups are important for maintaining heart health.

2.1 Understanding the Causes of Menopausal Symptoms

While changing hormone levels are a significant factor in menopausal symptoms, the NHAS's extensive research indicates that choices of lifestyle and nutritional imbalances also play a substantial role in symptom severity. Poor dietary habits, malabsorption, pregnancy, and breastfeeding can contribute to overall health depletion as menopause approaches.

2.2 Navigating the Menopausal Transition

Menopause often coincides with a period of significant mental and life changes, including concerns about aging, the future, and personal responsibilities. These additional stressors can compound the challenges of managing menopause symptoms. However, it is crucial to maintain perspective and recognize that menopause marks the beginning of a new phase that can be equally fulfilling. By addressing various contributing factors, you can ease the transition and minimize symptoms.

2.3 Determining Menopausal Status

Irregular periods or a prolonged absence of menstruation may indicate the onset of menopause. To ascertain menopausal status, two methods can be employed: requesting a test from a physician or conducting a home test. The home test measures follicle-stimulating hormone (FSH) levels in urine, which significantly increase during menopause. Consistently elevated FSH levels indicate menopause.

2.4 Types of Symptoms

Menopausal symptoms fall into three main categories:

- Signs of estrogen withdrawal: Night sweats, hot flashes, urinary symptoms, and sexual discomfort.

- Physical signs: Muscle aches, headaches, fatigue, constipation, and irritable bowel syndrome.

- Mental/emotional symptoms: Anxiety, mood swings, depression, confusion, and memory loss.

2.5 Managing Menopausal Symptoms

Women experiencing menopausal symptoms can explore various treatment options, including:

- Hormone replacement therapy (HRT): Temporary substitution of hormones like estrogen to alleviate symptoms.

- Vaginal estrogen: Used to increase lubrication and address vaginal dryness.

- Antidepressants: Can help alleviate low mood symptoms and improve hot flashes.

Additionally, adopting behavioral changes and self-care techniques can help reduce symptoms:

- Avoiding triggers like alcohol, spicy foods, and caffeine that can worsen hot flashes.

- Quitting smoking.

- Dressing in layers for easy cooling during hot flashes.

- Carrying cleansing wipes for freshening up on the go.

- Engaging in regular exercise for weight management, stress relief, and mood enhancement.

- Practicing relaxation techniques.

Chapter 3: What Changes Occur?

When the ovaries enter a phase of decreased hormone production, the conventional transformations associated with "menopause" take place. The ovaries, responsible for housing and releasing eggs, also play a role in producing progesterone and estrogen. These hormones work in harmony to regulate menstrual cycles and have an impact on blood cholesterol levels and calcium utilization within the body.

As menopause approaches, the final menstrual period occurs due to the cessation of egg production by the ovaries. Before reaching menopause, various physical changes manifest in the body, collectively referred to as "perimenopause," indicating a transition period. Alterations in the rhythm of menstrual periods are often the initial indicators of these changes. Periods may become irregular, heavier, shorter, longer, or even lighter in certain instances. The unpredictability of perimenopause can add uncertainty to one's life, along with potential mood swings, increased "black" days, and worsened premenstrual syndrome symptoms.

Additional symptoms include:

- Hot flashes

- Night sweats

- Mood changes

- Decreased libido

- Reduced energy levels

- Restless nights

- Trouble focusing

- Bladder control issues

- Sleep disturbances and emotional distress

- Managing concurrent medical conditions and medications

During the menopausal transition and beyond, estrogen levels decline, disrupting the typical cyclical rhythms of estrogen and progesterone in the body. Declining estrogen levels can significantly impact metabolism, potentially leading to weight gain and affecting cholesterol levels and carbohydrate digestion. Many women experience menopausal symptoms during this transition, including hot flashes and sleep disturbances.

Moreover, hormonal fluctuations contribute to a decrease in bone density, increasing the risk of fractures. Fortunately, dietary adjustments can help alleviate menopausal symptoms.

3.1 How These Changes Affect Different Aspects of the Body

Hormonal changes during menopause, particularly the decrease in progesterone and estrogen levels, significantly impact various areas of the female body. These changes may include:

- Modifications in menstrual cycles: Menstrual cycles leading up to menopause may become irregular, shorter, longer, heavier, or lighter until menstruation eventually ceases.

- Night sweats and hot flashes: Sudden sensations of heat, often accompanied by sweating, are characteristic signs of menopause. Hot flashes can disrupt sleep patterns and vary in frequency and intensity.

- Vaginal and urinary changes: Declining estrogen levels can lead to vaginal dryness, thinning, and reduced elasticity, resulting in discomfort, itching, and pain during sexual activity. The bladder and urinary system may also be affected, increasing the risk of urinary incontinence and urinary tract infections.

- Loss of bone density: The decline of estrogen during menopause heightens the risk of fractures and osteoporosis, making postmenopausal women more susceptible to bone-related disorders.

- Lipid profile changes: Menopause is associated with negative alterations in lipid profiles, including an increase in low-density lipoprotein (LDL) cholesterol and a decrease in high-density lipoprotein (HDL) cholesterol. These changes may elevate the risk of developing coronary artery disease.

- Mood changes: Hormonal fluctuations during menopause can impact emotions and mood, leading to mood swings, anger, anxiety, and feelings of sadness in some women.

- Sleep disruptions: Hot flashes, night sweats, and hormonal shifts can interfere with sleep patterns, causing insomnia or restless sleep. This can affect overall well-being and contribute to daytime fatigue.

- Metabolism changes: Menopause is linked to a decreased metabolic rate, potentially resulting in weight gain, particularly in the abdominal region. It can also alter fat storage patterns, increasing the risk of developing visceral fat.

- Skin and hair changes: Estrogen supports collagen production and skin elasticity. With its decline, women may experience drier skin, thinning skin, and an increased risk of wrinkles. Hair may also become drier and thinner.

- Cognitive changes: Some women report memory lapses, difficulties with focus, and changes in cognitive function during menopause. These changes are typically mild and may be influenced by hormone fluctuations and other factors.

Chapter 4: The Importance of Good Nutrition during This Sensitive Period

Nutritional practices are essential for supporting health and adjusting to the postmenopausal era since they include various issues that pertain to all women. These behaviors may be changed and significantly influence the quality of life and longevity. This review examines the available data on the relationship between dietary habits and important medical results in postmenopausal women, such as physique, bone density, and cardiovascular disease risk factors. According to the available research, switching to a low-fat, plant-based diet may improve one's body composition. However, further research is required to confirm these results, particularly in postmenopausal women. During the postmenopausal stage, avoiding bone, metabolism, and cardiovascular illnesses may be feasible by adopting a Mediterranean-style diet and implementing other healthy activities. This eating regimen, which strongly emphasizes items with soothing and antioxidant qualities, has been linked to moderate but substantial decreases in blood pressure, body fat mass, and cholesterol levels. However, further research is needed to determine the long-term impacts of these dietary decisions, particularly their influence on outcomes like bone fractures, obesity, and coronary ischemia.

Our diet has a significant influence on the variety and intensity of our symptoms of menopause. Interestingly, Asian women experience menopause differently than Western women. They don't often have hot flashes or night sweats, and until recently, the word "hot flush" didn't even exist in the Japanese language. The quantity of plant estrogens, or phytoestrogens, consumed by Westerners and Asians differs significantly.

Numerous studies conducted in recent years have shown that frequent use of estrogen-like substances throughout the day might be beneficial in a menopausal management program, much like HRT. Although having only around 1/1000th the potency of animal-based estrogen, phytoestrogens are rapidly gaining recognition as powerful hormone regulators due to their balanced effects on estrogen levels. Here is how they function. Phytoestrogens compete with estrogen for cell receptor sites when there is an excess of estrogen in the body, which can occur in women of adulthood. Receptors are structures on the surface of cells that allow hormonal substances and other substances into cells, much like a key opens a lock. Some phytoestrogens unavoidably replace estrogen and, due to the hormone's considerably lesser effects, may aid in reducing its ability to promote cancer.

Conversely, phytoestrogens may naturally increase your estrogen levels when they decline around menopause and beyond. According to research, a diet high in phytoestrogens, together with supplements and methods of relaxation, may help with menopausal symptoms as well as boost memory, cognitive performance, and heart health. Additionally, phytoestrogens could aid in osteoporosis prevention.

After controlling for other variables like age, weight, height, number of years since menopause, smoking, and everyday calcium intake, a study involving 650 women between the ages of nineteen and eighty-six discovered that postmenopausal women in the greatest amounts of dietary these compounds had a significantly greater density of bone minerals in their teeth and hips compared to those in the lowest intakes.

Soy milk, soybeans, tofu, soy flour, soy nuts, beans and lentils, chickpeas, mung beans, alfalfa, and red clover are all sources of isoflavones.

Lignans, green and yellow vegetables, flaxseeds, sesame seeds, sunflower seeds, pumpkin seeds, and almonds.

Menopausal symptoms may be managed with the use of two specific phytoestrogens.

They are lignans, found in flaxseeds, and isoflavones, present in red clover and soy products. The container on the left displays other sources of lignans and isoflavones. The typical daily intake of isoflavones in traditional Japanese foods ranges from 50 to 100 mg, but it is now less than 3 mg in the West.

Surprisingly, males may also benefit from a diet rich in isoflavones. Due to their diet's high isoflavone content, scientists think Asian men have a lower mortality rate from prostatic cancer and heart disease.

You should try consuming 100 mg of these compounds daily to help with menopausal symptoms. Given that isoflavones seem to leave the body somewhat fast, the best way to ensure you receive enough is to eat little phytoestrogen-rich foods often throughout the day.

Foods high in phytoestrogens are generally accessible and include soy yogurt and milk. According to estimates, flaxseeds contain around 300 times the amount of lignans than sunflower seeds.

When increasing your dietary intake of phytoestrogens, it's critical to take action to increase their absorption.

It's been established that an antibiotic course may also interfere with estrogen absorption for many months. Alcohol and cigarettes also tend to impair estrogen absorption. Improved phytoestrogen absorption may be achieved by limiting alcohol intake, reducing cigarette smoking, and taking a probiotic supplement following antibiotic treatment.

Your objective should be to eat a generally healthy diet and to replace some of the elements that nature and time have taken away, such as magnesium, zinc, B vitamins, and vital fatty acids, as well as ingesting 100mg of phytoestrogens daily. For the most important menopausal diet dos and don'ts, see dietary fat, hormones, and fiber.

Our Stone Age predecessors' diets are considerably different from those of today. Vegetable stuff, such as tough seeds and plant fiber like roots and stems, comprised most of their diet more than three million years ago, as opposed to the substantial quantities of animal protein we eat now. In addition, compared to the wild meat our ancestors consumed, the meat we purchase from butchers or supermarkets is substantially higher in fat, particularly saturated fat. According to research, your hormones are significantly impacted by the quantity of fat or fiber you consume.

Your likelihood of having high amounts of estrogen flowing in your body increases if your food is heavy in animal fat and low in fiber, which is common in the West. Your circulating estrogen levels will be lower if you follow a low-fat, high-fiber diet since dietary fiber positively affects how quickly estrogen departs the body.

Therefore, estrogen withdrawal may cause menopausal symptoms to occur considerably more often in Western women with high-fat, low-fiber diets. They respond to a rather high concentration of estrogen in the blood. Consequently, they are less able to withstand the menopausal decline in estrogen than women who have continuously had low levels of circulation estrogen throughout their lives.

This implies that switching drastically from your diet to a diet that is low in fat might worsen the effects of estrogen withdrawal. However, this effect is likely mitigated by the fact that your food is healthier, which, in turn, has a beneficial impact on how well your hormones are functioning. Do it gradually if you decide to alter your diet. Don't, for instance, abruptly go from a meat-eating lifestyle to a vegan one if you want to lose weight.

Chapter 5: The Recommended Foods and Why to Take Them

Optimal nutrition is crucial at every stage of life. When you maintain a healthy diet that includes a well-balanced mix of essential nutrients from various food groups and stay adequately hydrated, your body and mind receive energy and support to perform essential functions, leading to an improved quality of life.

As we approach middle age and women experience menopause, the importance of our dietary choices becomes even more significant. Hormonal changes and the natural aging process increase the demands on our bodies, making it essential to prioritize our nutrient intake. In this critical transitional period, the following section clearly outlines your nutritional requirements, emphasizing the importance of consuming the right amounts from each food group, avoiding certain foods, and highlighting the numerous benefits of healthy eating and the abundance of micronutrients they provide for both body and mind during the menopause years.

While some aging and menopause-related risk factors and symptoms are inevitable, adopting a proper diet can help prevent or alleviate certain diseases that may arise during or after menopause.

Many menopausal women experience muscle mass loss and a slower metabolism. According to a licensed dietitian and health coach, women going through menopause require less energy than when they were younger, making portion control the primary recommendation for women in this age group.

The National Institute of Health on Aging suggests that although you may need to consume fewer calories, it is crucial to ensure you still receive adequate vitamins and minerals to prevent conditions like osteoporosis and coronary artery disease. Therefore, choosing nutrient-dense meals becomes even more important. To ensure you meet all your body's nutritional needs, discussing dietary supplements with your healthcare provider or a registered dietitian nutritionist may be necessary. Additionally, selecting foods with therapeutic benefits specific to the menopausal phase of life can help alleviate symptoms.

It is advised to include a variety of foods in your diet to guarantee an appropriate intake of vital nutrients during menopause.

As iron and calcium are usually lacking in women's diets, it is advised to follow the following recommendations:

- Consume two to four servings of dairy goods and foods high in calcium daily (such as milk and yogurt, fish with bones, broccoli, and legumes). Attempt to consume 1,200 mg of calcium each day.

- Consume a minimum of three portions daily of iron-rich foods, such as lean red meat, chicken, fish, eggs, green leafy vegetables, nuts, and items made from enriched grains. For elderly women, a daily dose of 8 mg of iron is advised.

- Consume many high-fiber meals, including fresh fruits and vegetables, whole-grain cereals, breads, pasta, and rice. The average adult woman should aim for twenty-one grams of fiber each day.

- A minimum of one and a half cups of fruits and two cups of veggies should be consumed daily.

- Verify labels: Make healthier decisions by using the information on product labels.

- For adequate hydration, consume at least 8 glasses of water each day.

- Maintain an appropriate weight by limiting high-fat meals and reducing portion sizes if you are overweight. Speak with a licensed nutritionist or physician for advice on reaching a healthy weight.

- Limit high-fat foods: 25% to 35% of your daily calories should come from fat. Saturated fat, which may be found in animal products, and dairy products such as ice cream and cheese, should not make up more than 7% of your daily calorie intake. Limit your daily cholesterol consumption to 300 milligrams, and watch for Trans fats.

- Salt and sugar consumption should be kept in moderation to manage high blood pressure. Avoid eating foods smoked, salted, or charbroiled in large quantities because of their high nitrate content, which has been related to cancer.

- Limit your daily usage of alcohol to one drink or less.

5.1 Including Phytoestrogen in Your Diet Every Day

Here are some ideas on how to include phytoestrogens into your diet regularly.

- A sandwich prepared from two pieces of soy- and flaxseed-based bread. 22 mg of phytoestrogens are present.

- A 125 g/4 1/2 oz/1/2 cup serving of whipped soy dessert. 20 mg of phytoestrogens are present.

- A portion of 125 g/4 1/2 oz/1/2 cup soy yogurt. 10 mg of phytoestrogens are present.

- A 9 oz glass of soya fruit shake. 20 mg of phytoestrogens are present.

- A 9 oz glass of soy milk. 20 mg of phytoestrogens are present.

- Any Part 2 recipe that calls for 100 g/3 1/2 oz of tofu. 25 mg of phytoestrogens are present.

- A piece of flaxseed- and soy-based fruit loaf. 10 mg of phytoestrogens are present.

- A Phyto-Fix bar (page 191). 10 mg of phytoestrogens are present.

- Two vegan crepes. 10 mg of phytoestrogens are present.

- A serving of Phyto Muesli with soybean milk and flaxseeds that have been ground (see page 74). 30 mg of phytoestrogen is present.

You may get flaxseeds in the ground and seeded form; if you purchase them in ground form, you can easily add them to your cereals, yogurt, soups, smoothies, and shakes.

- **Enhanced Yogurt:** Calcium and vitamin D-rich food that supports bone health and other body processes. It keeps the heart, the nerves, and the muscles functioning.

- **Lean protein:** is found in foods including chicken, turkey, seafood, legumes, and lentils. Prolong your sense of fullness, lowering your risk of eating too much and gaining weight.

- Vital for maintaining muscular mass, particularly while participating in an exercise routine.

- **Salmon:** Rich in good fats and omega-3 fatty acids, which help elevate mood and lessen inflammation. Mood fluctuations related to menopause may be easier to control with omega-3s. Protein and the B12 vitamin are good energy sources and help control the neurotransmitters that affect our moods.

- **Water:** Since our bodies need regular replenishment, hydration is essential. Low energy levels brought on by dehydration might exacerbate menopausal symptoms. Hydration promotes general well-being and fights weariness.

- **Spinach:** A superb source of magnesium, it helps to regulate blood pressure, muscle and nerve function, and protein production.

- Lack of magnesium is linked to tension, anxiety, and difficulty unwinding. Including magnesium in your diet may promote relaxation and reduce insomnia symptoms.

- **Almonds:** Packed with fiber and protein, they help you feel satisfied and assist your digestive system. Magnesium and calcium are both good sources, which are good for bone health. Mild hot flashes may be relieved by the vitamin E in almonds.

- **Quinoa:** is a whole grain that contains magnesium, B vitamins, fiber, and protein. Superior to typical grains in terms of nutrients and gluten-free. Owing to its protein and fiber content, it gives fullness.

- **Omega-3 fatty acids:** Superior vitamins, minerals, and protein are all found in fish, which should be consumed at least eight ounces each week. Regular fish eating, particularly fatty fish like tuna and salmon, may lessen the likelihood of developing depression and ease hot flashes. The consumption of fish is good for your heart and general wellness.

- **Yogurt:** A probiotic food that provides calcium and protein for bone health, yogurt with live cultures is a popular choice.

Yogurt contains probiotics that improve digestive health, help in calcium and magnesium absorption, and support bone health. Yogurt may help control the symptoms of insomnia and enhance sleep quality.

- **Beans:** Beans provide a variety of minerals, fiber, and plant-based protein. Beans, which are high in fiber, help control blood sugar levels and lower the risk of developing type 2 diabetes. Beans include the aminoacid tryptophan, which is linked to better mood and mental health, and magnesium.

- **Soy:** Foods made from soy, such as tofu, edamame, and soymilk, are excellent plant-based protein sources that also include phytoestrogens. Soy's phytoestrogens may help with menopausal hot flashes and nocturnal sweats. Soy meals provide a wide range of gourmet possibilities and nutritional advantages.

- **Nuts:** Plant-based proteins, good fats, fiber, and vitamins may be found in nuts, including walnuts and pistachios. Although high in fat, nuts may help with weight control when consumed in moderation since they are filling. Every nut variety has particular health advantages, with walnuts being linked to a lower risk for depressive disorders and heart disease.

Chapter 6: Foods to Avoid and Why?

Your food choices have a big influence on how you feel throughout this transitional period naturally. Even if you don't feel like yourself, evaluating your food and supplement regimen to support fluctuating hormones, control the body's temperature, manage mood, and maintain energy levels is important. You may improve your whole state of being by making mindful dietary choices.

We have developed a list of items to avoid and healthy alternatives for each to help you make educated selections.

- **Taking hot chocolate cold:** Drinks with a heated temperature, such as hot chocolate, might make menopausal symptoms worse, especially if you have hot flashes. Hot chocolate mixes also often have high sugar content and little nutritional benefit. Choose rich in nutrients, cold, whey milk with chocolate as an alternative. The vitamin D and calcium that menopausal women require to promote the growth of bones, which is a major health issue at this stage of life, are either naturally present in milk or are supplemented with them.

- **Alternatives to caffeine for consistent energy:** Caffeine, often present in coffee, may exacerbate menopausal symptoms, such as difficulty sleeping and vasomotor signs like sweating during the night and flashes of heat. Consider nicotinamide riboside as an alternative to caffeine if you're tired during menopause since it helps with cellular energy generation, metabolism, and mitochondrial function.

- **Donuts and other high-carbohydrate:** Handled and calorically packed meals may cause hormonal changes, erratic energy levels, weight gain, and an elevated risk of cardiovascular disease. Instead, choose nutrient-dense substitutes like oatmeal with added berries, cinnamon, and peanut butter, which offer protein and fiber and help control blood sugar levels.

- **Alternatives to spicy foods:** Spicy foods may trigger or exacerbate night sweats, hot flashes, and typical menopausal temperature-control problems. Even though spices may increase metabolism and help with weight control, their use may worsen menopausal symptoms. Without the heat, you can flavor your cuisine with other spices. Sage, Chives, Lemon, Sweet Basil, Dill, and Garlic. They provide a powerful flavor without making the body overheat.

- **Reducing alcohol for improved sleep:** Alcohol interferes with the generation of melatonin, the hormone that controls sleep-wake cycles. Menopause-related sleep issues include trouble getting asleep, difficulty remaining asleep, and frequent wakings that may worsen. Instead, you may order a Virgin Mojito, which is simple for the bartender to make and a wonderful treat. Without the hangover, it's a new and revitalizing take on the classic drink. Ask the server at the bar if they can smash a few fruits at the bottom of the glass and then top it with some club soda for a sober take on a summer spritz. To finish off this wonderful alcohol-free beverage, add a squeeze of lemon.

- **Selecting healthy fats:** Fish over Fatty Meat: Fatty meat might be bad for your heart, particularly when your estrogen levels are down throughout menopause. The two omega-3 fatty acids (DHA and EPA) found in fatty fish, such as albacore tuna, are beneficial because they can lower the risk of coronary artery disease. Regular eating of oily fish has been linked to a postponement of natural menopause, which lowers the risk of heart attack and stroke.

- **Processed foods:** It is best to emphasize foods as near their natural condition as possible when making dietary selections.

Foods that are intensively processed and generally packaged in sacks or plastic may be deficient in important nutrients. As a result, it is advised to restrict the intake of certain meals.

- **Refined carbs:** Refined carbs like noodles, rice (white), and potatoes. The growth may increase insulin resistance and lead to blood sugar surges, exacerbating hot flashes.

Brown rice is an example of a whole grain that is a better option since it has a reduced effect on the level of sugar in the blood and offers more nutrients. Additionally, because they might further disturb blood sugar balance, sweet foods like cookies, cakes, and candies should be consumed in smaller amounts.

Chapter 7: Does Sugar Make Symptoms Worse?

During menopause, it is important to pay attention to sugar intake due to its potential impact on health and well-being. As women go through this transitional period, hormonal changes and metabolic shifts can increase the risk of weight gain and the development of chronic conditions such as diabetes and heart disease. Excessive consumption of sugar and high-glycemic foods can contribute to these health issues. Moreover, sugar can also exacerbate common menopausal symptoms such as mood swings, fatigue, and hot flashes. By adopting a diet low in added sugars and focusing on whole, nutrient-dense foods, women can better manage their weight, support hormonal balance, and reduce the likelihood of developing complications associated with menopause. It is advisable to prioritize natural sources of sweetness, such as fruits, and be mindful of hidden sugars in processed foods and beverages. By making conscious choices about sugar consumption, women can support their overall health and well-being during the menopausal transition.

According to several studies, women with low-sugar diets are likely to have fewer menopausal symptoms than those with high-sugar intake. According to one research that tracked 6,000 women for 9 years, those with a diet high in sugar had a 20% greater chance of having hot flashes and nocturnal sweats than those with lower sugar consumption. Estrogen's contribution to this relationship may be explained.

Estrogen levels change significantly during perimenopause, which causes unpleasant symptoms, including hot flashes and nocturnal sweats. An increase in insulin levels brought on by a high sugar intake lowers the body's supply of an amino acid called Sex Hormonal Binding Globulin (SHBG). When it comes to controlling estrogen, SHBG is essential. Estrogen levels rise when SHBG levels fall. In essence, a diet heavy in sugar causes an increase in estrogen. Therefore, if you eat a lot of sugar, your estrogen levels, which already fluctuate, may experience more significant rises and dips, aggravating menopausal symptoms.

Sugar intake might be especially harmful because of the hormonal shifts during menopause. This is why rising blood sugar levels and lower estrogen and progesterone levels cause cells to become more susceptible to insulin, raising blood sugar levels.

The chance of acquiring diseases, including diabetes, coronary artery disease, and some malignancies, may rise due to this insulin resistance. Additionally, weight gain and weariness are linked to high blood sugar levels.

7.1 Hot Flashes and Sugar

Hot flashes, a typical menopausal symptom, have been linked to high blood sugar levels. Consuming sugary meals may result in blood sugar swings that exacerbate the occurrence and severity of hot flashes. Eating items with a low glycemic index, such as fruits and vegetables, grains, nuts, and milk and cheese, is crucial to maintain stable blood sugar levels.

7.2 HRT

Hormone Replacement Therapy Sugar and its effects on insulin may reduce the efficacy of HRT in menopausal women who take it to relieve symptoms. Excessive sugar consumption may exacerbate menopausal symptoms even in those not on HRT.

Given these factors, cutting down on sugar is strongly advised during menopause. It's crucial to remember that eliminating sugar may not be required. Positive outcomes may be attained by making little changes and switching to a healthier diet.

7.3 Guidelines for Cutting Sugar Intake

- **Verify labels:** Be diligent in looking for added sugars on food labels. To better manage the quantity of sugar in your diet, look for alternate brands or think about making meals from scratch.

- **Cook more:** Use the internet to research dishes and cooking techniques with low sugar content. You may alter ingredients and eliminate hidden sugars when you prepare your meals.

- **Learn more:** Learn about the impact of glucose and the advantages of a sugar-free diet. Read books, newspapers, TV programs, podcasts, and other trustworthy sources for insightful information.

- **Select real food:** Choose whole, unadulterated foods over manufactured ones, which often have sneaky sugars. Put healthful foods at the top of your priority list by purchasing fresh produce or signing up for a community-supported agriculture program.

- **Accept fruit:** Increase your consumption of fruit. Fruit contains natural sugars, fiber, and water, making them a healthier alternative to processed and added sweets. Eating various fruits to satisfy your sweet need while enjoying the fruits' nutritional advantages.

Reduced risk of coronary artery disease, type 2 diabetes, and specific cancers, simpler weight control, and higher food quality are just a few benefits of cutting less on sugar. Making thoughtful decisions and gradually cutting down on sugar will help you experience fewer blood sugar swings and perhaps lessen menopausal symptoms.

Chapter 8: Hydration

The process of ensuring that the body has a proper fluid balance is called hydration. Water is a key component of many physiological processes. Thus, it is crucial for general health and well-being. Due to the unique changes and difficulties connected with this time of life, maintaining appropriate hydration is even more crucial during menopause.

- **Temperature control:** Night sweats and hot flashes are common in menopausal women and may result in more sweat and fluid loss. Maintaining fluid balance helps control body temperature and manages these symptoms.

- **Hydrating results:** Dry skin, eyes, and nasal passages may be brought on by hormonal changes during menopause. Drinking enough water daily keeps the body hydrated, which may enhance skin suppleness, reduce dryness, and promote a healthy balance of moisture in the body. Infections of the urinary tract (UTIs) and bladder problems are more likely to occur after menopause. Enough water consumption lowers the risk of UTIs and improves bladder health by flushing out germs and chemicals from the urinary tract.

Dehydration may have a detrimental effect on bone health. As estrogen levels fall throughout menopause, the likelihood of fractures rises. Drinking enough water helps the body maintain healthy bone mineralization and fends against bone-related problems.

- **General satisfaction:** Water intake has to be right for general health and well-being. It supports the operation of the body's essential organs, facilitates digestion, increases energy, and fosters cognitive function. During menopause, staying hydrated may aid with tiredness relief, mood-lifting, and overall quality of life improvements.

Throughout the day, it is advised to drink enough water; aim for eight cups (64 ounces) or further, depending on personal requirements and activity levels. To maintain your health throughout menopause, it's crucial to pay attention to your body's thirst signals and make sure you're drinking enough fluids.

8.1 Why Is Enough Hydration Crucial During Menopause?

As a result of the major effects that menopause has on the body, maintaining appropriate hydration is essential. Here's why being hydrated is essential:

- **Essential purposes:** Every cell, tissue, and muscle in the body needs water to operate properly. It assists in elimination, circulates nutrients, speeds up metabolism, removes toxins, and enhances blood circulation. It also helps control body temperature.

- **Menopausal symptoms are affected:** Dehydration may intensify and increase the frequency of menopausal symptoms. Joint pain, dry skin, abdominal pain, constipation, migraines, brain fog, vitamin shortages, high blood pressure, night sweats, hot flashes, exhaustion, dry vaginal passages, and other problems might result from insufficient water.

- **Joint well-being:** Water is essential for lubricating the joints, encouraging fluid motion, and minimizing discomfort and inflammation.

- **Skin health:** Just as a grape plumps up compared to a raisin, proper hydration helps moisturize and nourish the skin, boosting its quality and reducing dryness.

- **Stomach health:** Getting enough water helps the body produce salivary and stomach acids, which aids in effective digestion and lessens symptoms like gas, abdominal pain, and inflammation. Water is necessary for healthy bowel movements and urine function, which helps the body eliminate toxins and waste. Bowel movements, slower

Elimination, and a higher likelihood of infections may result from insufficient water.

- **Blood flow:** Dehydration may reduce blood supply to the brain, causing migraines, foggy thinking, diminished memory, and mood disorders, including anxiety and melancholy. The brain is largely made of water. Optimal blood flow is supported by adequate hydration, ensuring the distribution of oxygen, minerals, and hormones throughout the body. Hot flushes, nocturnal sweats, exhaustion, and vitamin deficits may all be caused by not drinking enough water.

- **Sexual health:** Lack of hydration may lead to vaginal dryness and pain during everyday activities and sexual activity. Water helps supply moisture for lubricating the vaginal tube.

It is advised to consume a minimum of 2 liters of water per day, select a high-quality water source, avoid drinking too much salt, limit the amount of diuretic drinks like beverages, alcohol, and carbonated beverages, and track urine color as a measure of hydration levels. A nearby water container might also assist in replenishing fluids lost during nocturnal sweats.

Staying adequately hydrated is crucial during menopause to support overall health and manage certain symptoms associated with this life stage. Hormonal changes during menopause can lead to increased perspiration and hot flashcs, causing women to lose more water through sweating. Additionally, aging can affect the body's ability to regulate fluid balance. Menopausal women must prioritize hydration to prevent dehydration, support optimal bodily functions, and alleviate symptoms like hot flashes and dryness.

Drinking adequate water throughout the day helps maintain body temperature, supports cognitive function, promotes skin health, and aids digestion. It is recommended to consume at least 8 glasses (64 ounces) of water daily and even more if engaging in physical activity or spending time in hot environments. Along with water, herbal teas, and infused water can provide hydration while adding variety to the daily fluid intake. By prioritizing hydration, menopausal women can support their overall well-being and effectively manage symptoms associated with this stage of life.

Chapter 9: Dietary Supplements When Needed

In place of pharmaceutical hormones, which many women are reluctant to use to address menopausal symptoms, botanical and nutritional supplements (BDS) are becoming more popular. Although there is no scientific proof of these items' efficacy and long-term security, many women are drawn to these "natural therapies." Women in their premenopausal and postmenopausal stages are among those who use BDS products the most, although a sizable portion (70%) don't tell their doctors about it. Few doctors ask their patients about their use of BDS, mostly because they were not exposed to alternative medical methods throughout their training and have little experience with these items, exacerbating the problem. The typical botanicals and nutritional supplements used in menopause—such as red clover, black cohosh, for example, soybeans, and others—are examined in this review study.

9.1 Black Cohosh: A Hot Flash Cure?

One of the supplements for menopause that has been the subject of the most research is black cohosh, made from the roots of herbal plants.

When contrasted to a placebo, multiple studies have demonstrated its efficacy, especially in lowering vasomotor signs like hot flashes. However, some research has shown contradictory findings. It's crucial to remember that black cohosh shouldn't be used by those who have liver issues.

9.2 Eliminating Night Sweats with Flaxseed

Some women may relieve moderate menopausal symptoms by consuming flaxseed and flaxseed oil. These goods are abundant in lignans, which were recently discovered to assist in regulating female hormones. However, not every study has consistently shown how effective flaxseed is in reducing vasomotor symptoms like night sweats.

9.3 Calcium: Keeping Bones Strong

The drop in hormone levels after menopause may cause considerable bone loss. Getting enough calcium at this time is essential. Women under 51 need 1,000 mg of calcium daily, while those above 51 need 1,200. When feasible, it is best to get calcium via dietary sources. It is preferable to take supplements in smaller amounts during the day with meals (no over 500 milligrams at a time) to improve absorption.

9.4 Popular Yet with Little Support for Red Clover

Given that it includes natural plant estrogens, red clover is often utilized by women wanting relief from menopausal symptoms. However, study results on its efficacy have been conflicting. Recent research has not shown an elevated risk of uterus cancer linked to three months of red clover consumption. Nevertheless, a doctor should be consulted if there are any worries regarding its use.

9.5 Sunlight and Supplements for Vitamin D

Like calcium, vitamin D is essential for preserving bone health. The body cannot adequately absorb calcium without sufficient vitamin D. The average adult needs 600 international units of vitamin D per day, while those over 71 need 800 IU. In addition to particular meals and pills, sunshine is another way to get vitamin D. It is crucial to remember that even little sun exposure may cause skin damage. Therefore, it is best to depend mostly on food sources and consider taking supplements if necessary.

Dietary supplements can play a beneficial role in supporting women during menopause by addressing specific nutrient needs and alleviating associated symptoms.

Menopause is when hormonal fluctuations and physiological changes impact overall health and well-being.

Here are ways in which dietary supplements can be helpful during this stage:

- **Maintaining bone health:** Menopause is frequently accompanied by a reduction in bone density, elevating the susceptibility to osteoporosis. Enhancing bone health and mitigating the risk of fractures can be achieved through the utilization of calcium and vitamin D supplements.

- **Relieving menopausal symptoms:** Certain supplements, such as black cohosh, evening primrose oil, and soy isoflavones, have been studied for their potential to alleviate hot flashes, night sweats, mood swings, and other common menopausal symptoms. However, consulting with a healthcare professional before starting any new supplement regimen is important.

- **Supporting heart health:** Menopause is associated with an increased risk of cardiovascular disease. Omega-3 fatty acids, particularly from fish oil supplements, can help support heart health by reducing inflammation and maintaining healthy cholesterol levels.

- **Mood and sleep support:** Some women experience mood swings, irritability, and sleep disturbances during menopause. Supplements like St. John's wort, valerian root, and melatonin may promote better sleep quality and support emotional well-being.

- **Maintaining hormonal balance:** Certain herbal supplements, including red clover and dong quai, are believed to help balance hormones during menopause. However, more research is needed to fully understand their effectiveness and safety.

9.6 Supplements to Complete Your Nutritional Bases and Add to Your Support

While good eating is your best line of defense against aging, supplementing wisely may help you make sure you're meeting all of your nutritional needs and promoting healthy aging.

Multivitamin

A multivitamin-mineral complex formulated especially for women over 50 should be taken first. Look for an item that is low in iron or doesn't contain iron if you're no longer menstruating and hence not losing iron via blood loss.

The Fatty Acids Omega-3

At least eight ounces of fish should be consumed each week, according to the dietary recommendations for Americans. If you don't eat enough fish or don't eat it often enough to satisfy the recommendation, think about taking an omega-3 supplement or consuming oils rich in omega-3 fatty acids, such as flaxseed oil.

N-3 fatty acids are categorized as beneficial fats that can potentially alleviate menopausal symptoms. These essential fatty acids have shown to lower inflammation while improving the health of the heart and brain.

Medications that Reduce Inflammation

Even while irritation is a natural process that is vital for recuperation, when it persists for a long time, it may harm blood vessels, tissues, and joints. Alzheimer's, heart disease, and arthritis may all be brought on by this injury. A blood test measuring the liver enzyme known as C-reactive protein may be used to evaluate if you have chronic inflammation.

Several other supplements, in addition to fish oils, may help decrease inflammation:

Turmeric: Research suggests that the turmeric compound turmeric may lower C-reactive protein.

Consuming ginger, according to studies, may help lower C-reactive protein.

Resveratrol: When used as a supplement, this antioxidant, which is also present in purple foods like blueberries and grapes, has been demonstrated to lessen inflammation.

- **Spirulina:** Studies have also shown that the blue-green algae spirulina may lessen inflammation.

- **Vitamin C:** Vitamin C, a potent antioxidant, may help reduce inflammation.

Consult your doctor or qualified dietitian before taking a food supplement to reduce irritation and promote longevity, particularly if you are on medication or have a specific medical condition.

Chapter 10: Herbal Remedies for Menopausal Symptoms

Herbs have long been used as a natural approach to alleviating the symptoms of menopause. Several herbs have shown the potential to improve various menopausal symptoms. One such herb is black cohosh (Actaea racemosa), traditionally used to relieve hot flashes, mood swings, and sleep disturbances. Another herb, red clover (Trifolium pratense), contains isoflavones with estrogen-like effects, potentially reducing hot flashes and vaginal dryness. Dong quai (Angelica sinensis), an herb commonly used in traditional Chinese medicine, is believed to help regulate hormone levels and relieve menopausal symptoms. Additionally, evening primrose oil, derived from the evening primrose plant's seeds, is known for its potential benefits in reducing hot flashes and bone loss. While these herbs show promise, it is important to consult with a healthcare professional before incorporating them into a menopause management plan to ensure safety and appropriate usage.

- **Phytoestrogens:** Certain herbs contain compounds called phytoestrogens, which are plant-based substances that can mimic the effects of estrogen in the body. These compounds may help alleviate menopausal symptoms by providing a mild estrogenic effect and balancing hormone levels.

- **Mood regulation:** Some herbal remedies have properties that can help regulate mood and reduce symptoms of anxiety, irritability, and depression commonly experienced during menopause. These herbs may act on neurotransmitters and brain receptors involved in mood regulation.

- **Sleep improvement:** Certain herbs have sedative or calming properties that can promote better sleep and alleviate insomnia, a common symptom of menopause. These herbs may help relax the nervous system and induce a sense of calmness, facilitating restful sleep.

- **Anti-inflammatory effects:** Inflammation is believed to play a role in menopausal symptoms. Some herbal remedies possess anti-inflammatory properties that can help reduce inflammation, potentially alleviating symptoms such as hot flashes, joint pain, and muscle discomfort.

- **Adaptogenic effects:** Adaptogenic herbs can help the body adapt and respond to stress more effectively. Menopause is a period of hormonal changes that can lead to increased stress levels. Adaptogenic herbs help support the body's stress response and promote overall well-being during this transitional phase.

Some herbal remedies and lifestyle changes may reduce menopausal symptoms and help you feel more comfortable. There's also evidence that changing your diet can help with symptoms.

10.1 Herbs to Improve Symptoms of Menopause

Herbal remedies can potentially affect menopausal symptoms through various mechanisms. Here are some ways in which herbal remedies may have an impact:

For Hot Flashes/Night Sweats

- **Black Cohosh:** Black cohosh, derived from the root of the North American black cohosh plant, has been studied for its potential to reduce hot flashes and other menopause symptoms. While some studies suggest its efficacy, more research is needed for conclusive evidence.

- **Red Clover:** Red clover, containing natural plant estrogens, is commonly used for menopause symptom relief. However, research results are mixed, and further studies are necessary.

- **Soy:** Soy is a source of isoflavones, phytoestrogens, or plant estrogens. Some studies suggest that soy may help reduce menopausal symptoms. However, the findings could be more consistent, as other studies have shown no significant benefit.

Consuming soy in its food forms, such as tofu or soy milk, is recommended rather than in tablet or powder form.

- **Wild Yams:** Studies on wild yam cream have yielded mixed results for menopause symptom relief. Research on a protein found in wild purple yams is limited to animal studies, requiring further investigation.

For Bone Loss/Hot Flashes

- **Evening primrose (Oenothera biennis):** Indigenous to central and eastern North America, this blossoming plant is known for its seed oil, which is commonly employed as a natural remedy for alleviating menopause symptoms such as hot flashes and bone loss.

To evaluate the efficacy of the supplement in alleviating hot flashes, a 2013 clinical trial administered oral Evening Primrose Oil (EPO) for six weeks, comparing it to a placebo. The study demonstrated a decrease in the intensity of hot flashes and, to a lesser degree, in their frequency and duration.

For Sexual Health/Hot Flashes

- **Licorice:** Licorice root has shown promise in relieving hot flashes and improving sexual health.

- It is important to note that consuming large amounts of licorice could lead to negative side effects, so consulting with a healthcare professional is advised.

- **Anise:** Anise may help reduce the frequency and severity of hot flashes, although more research is needed to establish its effectiveness.

For Mental & Personal Health

- **Fennel:** Fennel has been studied for its potential benefits in mental health and addressing vaginal atrophy during menopause. However, further investigation is required to confirm its effectiveness.

- **Ginseng:** Ginseng root has been associated with potential improvements in sex drive, hot flashes, and symptoms of depression in menopausal women. Additional high-quality studies are needed for stronger evidence.

- **Maca Root:** Limited research suggests that maca root may enhance sex drive in menopausal women, particularly those taking antidepressants. Further studies are required for conclusive evidence.

For Insomnia Problem

- **Valerian:** scientifically known as Valeriana officinalis, is an herbal remedy available as tea or tablets derived from the plant's root and rhizome. It has been found to aid insomnia treatment by enhancing sleep quality, particularly in postmenopausal women. However, it may require consistent use for up to four weeks before noticeable effects are observed.

For Vaginal Dryness

- **Black Cohosh:** Black cohosh, derived from the root of the North American black cohosh plant, has been studied for its potential to reduce vagina dryness and other menopausal symptoms.

For Mood Problems

- **St. John's wort:** It is a traditional herbal remedy for addressing mild to moderate symptoms of anxiety, irritability, and depressed mood commonly associated with menopause.

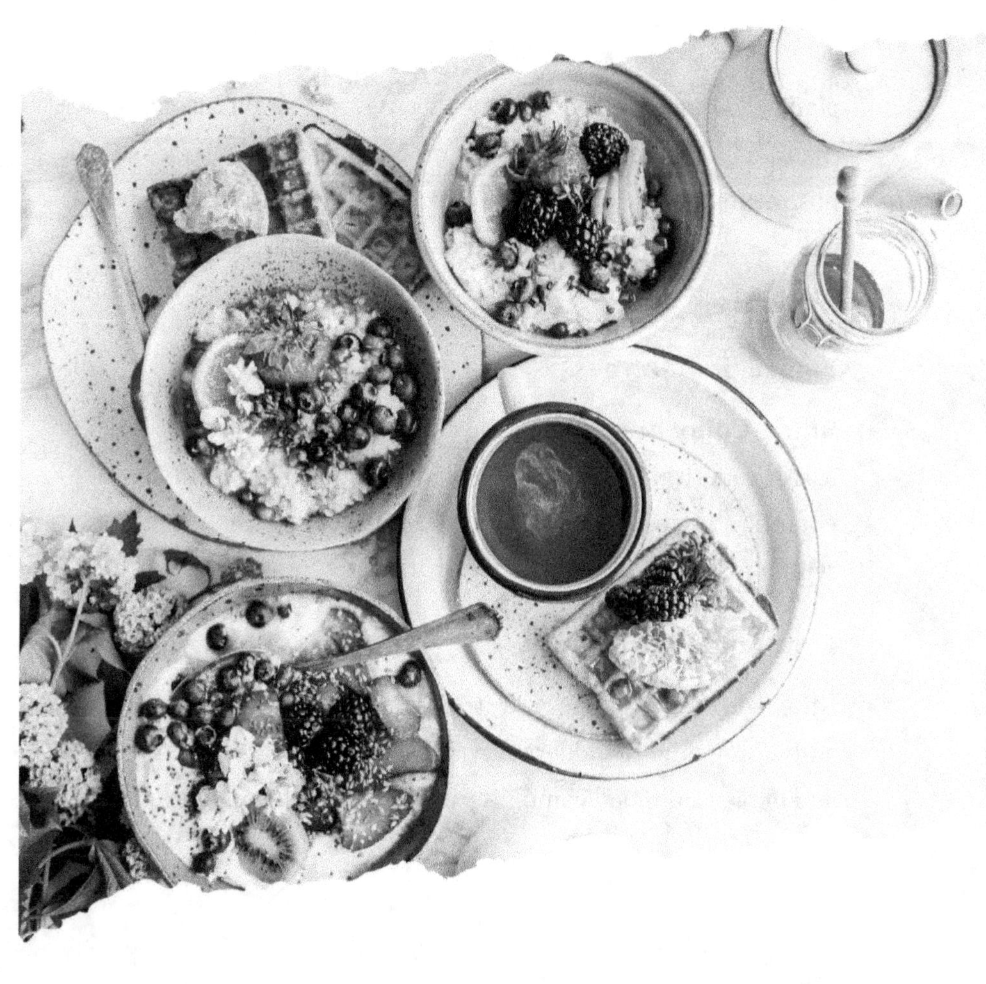

Chapter 11: Hormone Healing 100 Recipes

Breakfast Recipes

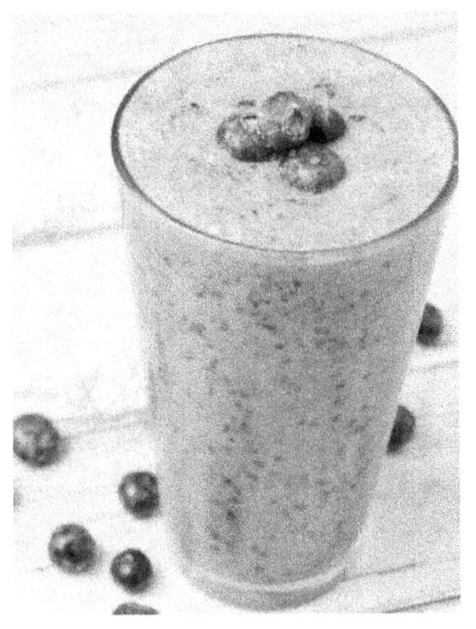

Rhubarb & Blueberry Smoothie

  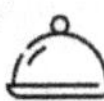

Prep Time	Cook Time	Servings
5 min	15 min	2

Method:

INGREDIENTS:

- 3 tbsp hone
- ¼ tsp vanilla
- extract
- 1 ½ cups blueberries
- 2 cups chilled soy milk
- 8 oz/1 ¾ cups trimmed

& chopped rhubarb

- 8 ice cubes to serve

1. Preheat the oven to 200°C/400°F/Gas 6.

2. Place the rhubarb on a baking sheet and drizzle it with honey.

3. Roast the rhubarb in the oven for about 15 minutes or until it becomes tender. Once done, set it aside to cool.

4. Combine the roasted rhubarb, blueberries, chilled soy milk, honey, and vanilla extract in a blender or food processor.

NUTRITIONAL

VALUE:

- Calories: 216
- Carbohydrates:

33.8 g

- Protein: 8.1 g
- Fat: 4.7 g

5. Blend the ingredients until you achieve a smooth and creamy consistency.

6. Serve the smoothie immediately. Optionally, add ice cubes to enhance its chill facto

7.

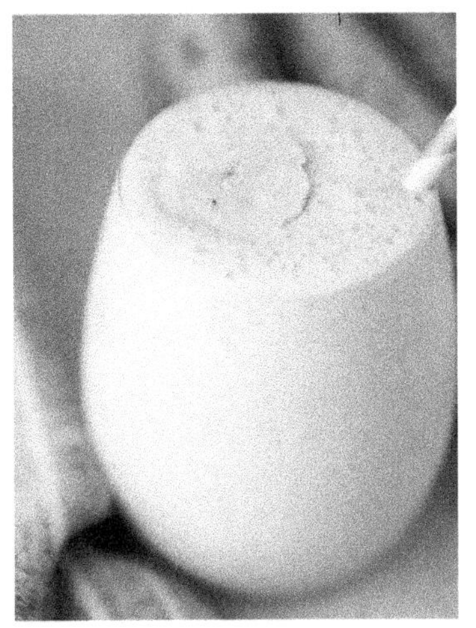

Banana Shake

Prep Time	Cook Time	Servings
5 min	15 min	2

INGREDIENTS:

- 2 ripe bananas
- ¼ tsp ground nutmeg
- ¼ cup ground almonds
- 2 cups chilled soy milk

Method:

1. Peel the ripe bananas and place them in a blender or food processor.

2. Add the ground almonds, nutmeg, and chilled soy milk to the blender.

3. Blend all the ingredients until smooth and creamy.

4. Transfer the shake to the refrigerator and let it chill for about 15 minutes.

NUTRITIONAL VALUE:

- Calories: 242
- Carbohydrates: 27.5 g
- Protein: 10.7 g
- Fat: 10.1 g

5. Serve the banana shake immediately.

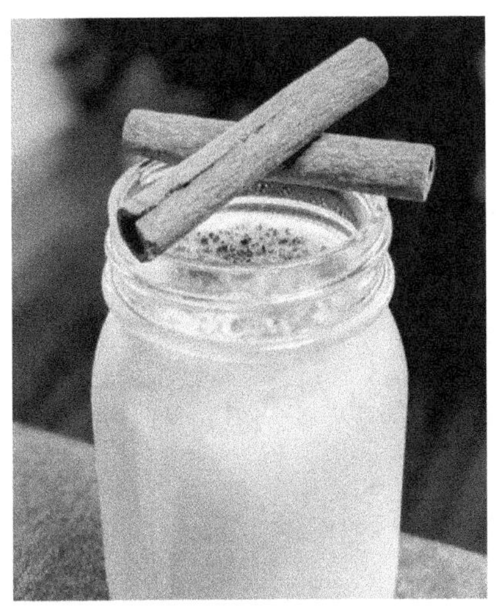

Honey & Cinnamon

Soy Milk

Prep Time   Cook Time   Servings

5 min   15 min   2

Method:

INGREDIENTS:

- 3 tbsp hone
- ¼ tsp vanilla extract
- 1 ½ cups blueberries
- 2 cups chilled soy milk
- 8 oz/1 ¾ cups trimmed

& chopped rhubarb

- 8 ice cubes to serve

1. Preheat the oven to 200°C/400°F/Gas 6.

2. Place the rhubarb on a baking sheet and drizzle it with honey.

3. Roast the rhubarb in the oven for about 15 minutes or until it becomes tender. Once done, set it aside to cool.

4. Combine the roasted rhubarb, blueberries, chilled soy milk, honey, and vanilla extract in a blender or food processor.

NUTRITIONAL VALUE:

- Calories: 216
- Carbohydrates:

33.8 g

- Protein: 8.1 g
- Fat: 4.7 g

5. Blend the ingredients until you achieve a smooth and creamy consistency.

6. Serve the smoothie immediately. Optionally, add ice cubes to enhance its chill factor is desired

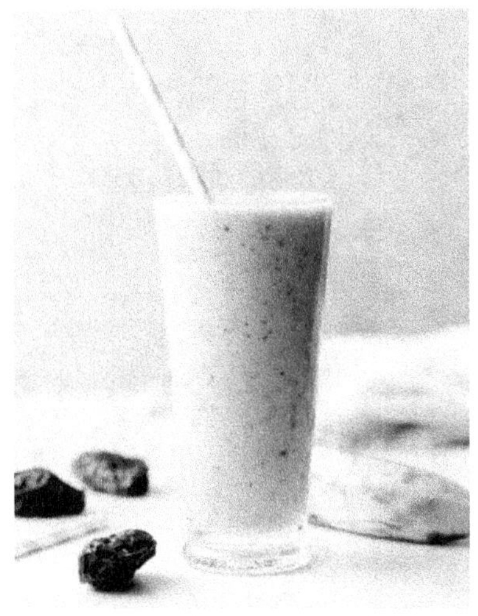

Creamy Banana

Date Shake

Prep Time	Cook Time	Servings
5 min	15 min	2

Method:

1. Place the silken tofu, ripe banana, pitted dates, and apple juice in a blender or food processor.

2. Blend all the ingredients until they become smooth and creamy.

3. Serve the creamy banana and date shake immediately.

4. Optionally, add ice cubes to the shake for a refreshing touch.

INGREDIENTS:

- 4 pitted dates
- 1 ¾ oz silken tofu
- 1 very ripe banana, small
- ⅓ cup apple juice
- 8 ice cubes to serve
-

NUTRITIONAL

VALUE:

- Calories: 98
- Carbohydrates: 18.3 g
- Protein: 3.1 g
- Fat: 1.5 g

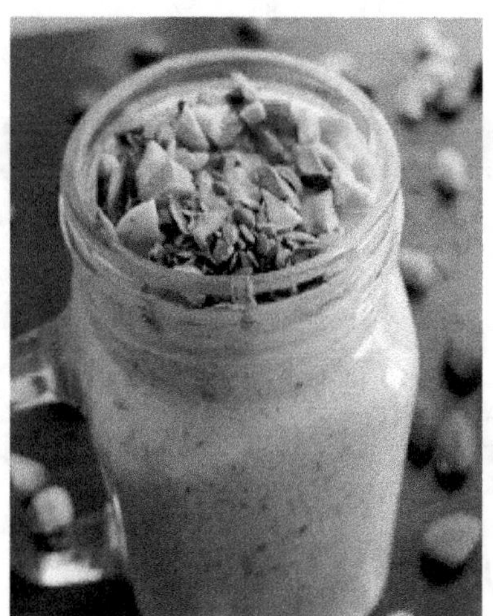

Creamy Banana

Date Shake

Prep Time	Cook Time	Servings
5 min	15 min	2

INGREDIENTS:

- 4 pitted dates
- 3 pieces fruit, peeled & chopped (e.g., 1 mango, 1 pear, and 1 apple)
- ¼ cup ground almonds or golden flaxseeds
- 2 cups plain yogurt
- 8 ice cubes to serve

NUTRITIONAL VALUE:

- Calories: 255
- Carbohydrates: 19.6 g
- Protein: 11.4 g
- Fat: 14.6 g
-

Method:

1. Place the chopped pieces of fruit, ground almonds or golden flaxseeds, plain yogurt, and ice cubes (if desired) in a blender or food processor.

2. Blend all the ingredients until they are smooth and creamy.

3. Serve the fruit and nut shake immediately.

4. Optionally, add ice cubes to the shake for an extra chilled

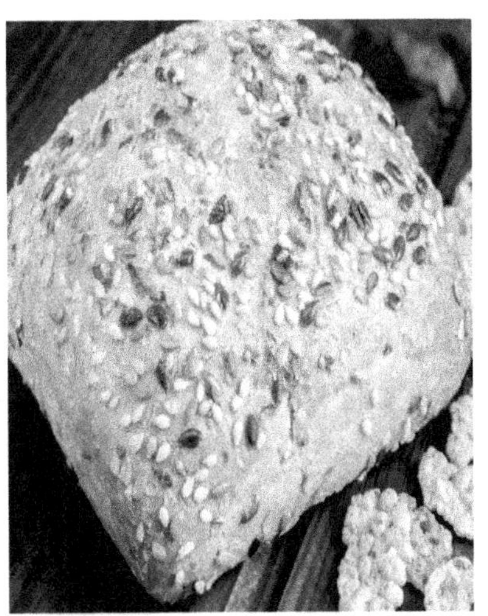

Phyto Fruit Loaf

Prep Time	Cook Time	Servings
1 hr. 10 min	1 hr. 15 min	8

INGREDIENTS:

- ½ heaped cups soy flour
- ½ cup buckwheat flour
- 1/8 cup flaxseeds
- 1/8 cup ground almonds
- ⅓ cup sesame seeds
- 2 ¼ cups dried fruit

(such as raisins, currants,

apricots)

- 2 tbsp unrefined

caster/superfine \sugar

- 1 tsp ground nutmeg
- 1 tsp mixed/apple pie spice
- 1 tbsp cinnamon

Method:

In a large mixing bowl, sift the soy flour and buckwheat flour. Stir in the flaxseeds, ground almonds, sesame seeds, sunflower seeds, dried fruit, sugar, nutmeg, mixed/apple pie spice, cinnamon, and grated ginger.

2. Pour in the soy milk and mix thoroughly to create a dough. Cover the bowl with cling film/plastic wrap and let it stand at room temperature for 1 hour.

85

2 pieces, root ginger, grated

- 2 tsp baking powder
- 3 ½ cups scant soy milk
- Sunflower oil for

greasing

- For serving: butter,

cheese,

peanut butter, or

sugar-free jam

Nutritional Value:

- Calories: 183
- Carbohydrates: 20.8 g
- Protein: 8.9 g
- Fat: 7.3 g

3. Preheat the oven to 350°F/Gas 4 and grease a 2 lb loaf tin with sunflower oil.

4. Spoon the dough mixture into the prepared loaf tin, spreading it evenly.

5. Bake in the preheated oven for about 1 hour and 15 minutes or until the top is firm and golden.

6. Remove from the oven and let it cool in the tin for 5 minutes, then transfer to a wire rack to cool completely.

7. Serve the fruit loaf sliced, either warm or cooled, and enjoy it with butter, cheese, peanut butter, or sugar-free jam.

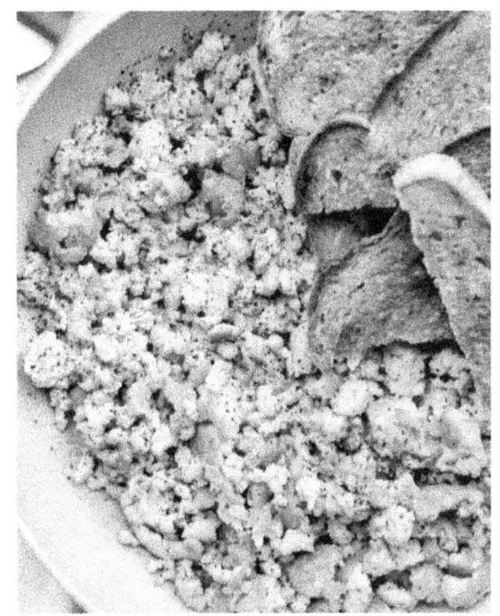

INGREDIENTS:

- 1 tbsp soy oil
- 1 small onion, finely

chopped

- 1 carrot, finely

chopped

- 1 potato, diced
- 4 cups diced tofu
- 1 ½ tsp turmeric
- ½ tsp black pepper

Scrambled Tofu

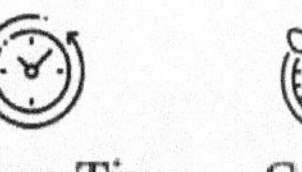  

Prep Time	Cook Time	Servings
15 min	25 min	4

Method:

1. Heat soy oil in a large frying pan over low heat. Add the finely chopped onion and cook, stirring occasionally, for 2-3 minutes or until golden.

2. Add the finely chopped carrot and diced potato to the pan. Cook, stirring frequently, for another 10 minutes or until they are slightly soft.

3. Stir in the diced tofu, turmeric, and black pepper. Cover the pan with a lid and cook for 5 minutes,

For serving:

- 2 tomatoes, halved
- 4 mushrooms
- 4 slices toasted rye

bread

Nutritional Value:

- Calories: 413
- Carbohydrates:

26.5 g

- Protein: 27.3 g
- Fat: 20 g

allowing the mixture to heat through and absorb the flavors.

4. Meanwhile, preheat the grill/broiler to medium. Place the halved tomatoes and mushrooms under the grill/broiler for 6-7 minutes or until their tops are slightly golden.

5. Serve the scrambled tofu hot, accompanied by the grilled tomatoes, mushrooms, and toasted rye bread.

6. In a large mixing bowl, sift the soy flour and buckwheat flour. Stir in the flaxseeds, ground almonds, sesame seeds, sunflower seeds, dried fruit, sugar, nutmeg, mixed/apple pie spice, cinnamon, and grated ginger.

7. Pour in the soy milk and mix thoroughly to create a dough. Cover the bowl with cling film/plastic wrap and let it stand at room temperature for 1 hour

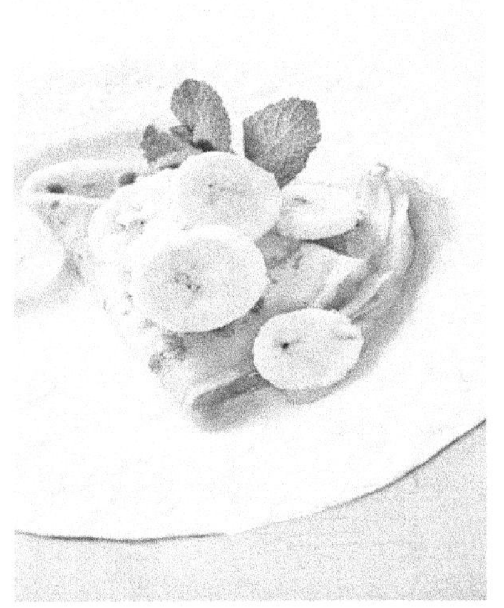

Banana Oat Crepes

Prep Time	Cook Time	Servings
15 min	15 min	4

INGREDIENTS:

- ½ cup rolled oats
- ½ cup soy flour
- 1 tbsp rice flour
- 1 tbsp baking powder
- 1 cup unsweetened soy milk
- 2 thinly sliced bananas
- 1 tbsp sunflower oil

Method:

1. Combine the rolled oats, soy flour, rice flour, and baking powder in a large mixing bowl. Create a well in the center and pour in the soy milk. Use a wooden spoon to beat the mixture until it forms a smooth batter. Add the thinly sliced bananas and gently stir until well-mixed. Cover the bowl and let the batter stand for at least 10 minutes, or refrigerate for 30 minutes.

2. Heat a large non-stick frying pan over medium heat until hot. Add

For serving:

- Maple syrup
- Soy yogurt
- Fruit

Nutritional Value:

- Calories: 356
- Carbohydrates:

32.3 g

- Protein: 20.7 g
- Fat: 16 g

half the sunflower oil and tilt the pan to ensure the bottom is completely coated with oil. Pour 2 tablespoons of the batter into the pan and tilt it to spread the mixture evenly over the bottom. Cook for approximately 2 minutes until bubbles appear on the surface, then use a spatula to turn the crêpe. Cook for an additional minute or until the bottom is slightly golden. Transfer the cooked crêpe to a plate.

3. Repeat the process with the remaining batter, adding more oil to the pan until all the batter has been used.

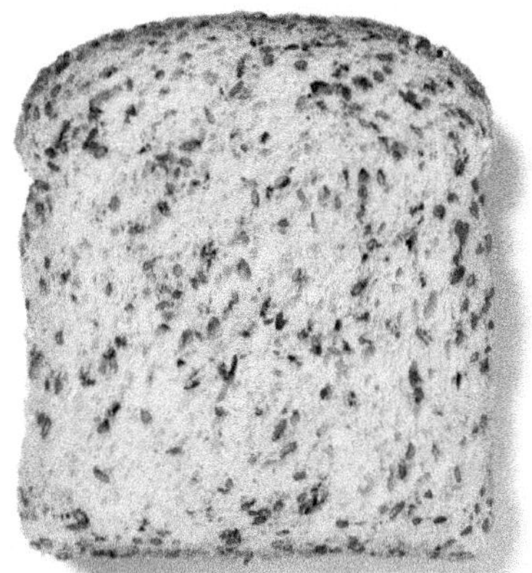

Sussex Soy Bread

Prep Time	Cook Time	Servings
10 min	50 min	5

Method:

INGREDIENTS:

- 3 eggs
- 3 tbsp walnut oil
- ¾ cup soy flour
- ½ cup maize flour
- ¾ cup heaped rice flour
- 2 tbsp soft light brown

sugar

- 2 tbsp Phyto Sprinkle

(or your preferred

seasonin blend)

1. Preheat the oven to 180°C/350°F/Gas 4 and grease a 900g/2lb loaf pan with sunflower oil.

2. Sift the soy flour, maize flour, rice flour, sugar, Phyto Sprinkle, yeast, and baking powder into a food processor. Add the walnut oil and blend until well combined.

3. In a separate bowl, whisk together the eggs and soy milk. Pour the egg mixture into the food processor and blend until the batter is smooth.

- 1 ½ tsp fast-action dried yeast

- 2 heaped tsp baking powder

- 1 cup unsweetened soy milk

For greasing

- Sunflower Oil

Nutritional Value:

- Calories: 384

- Carbohydrates: 35.6 g

- Protein: 17.1 g

- Fat: 18.2 g

4. Spoon the batter into the greased loaf pan, spreading it evenly.

5. Bake in the oven for 50 minutes or until the bread is golden brown and a toothpick inserted into the center comes clean.

6. Remove from the oven and let it cool in the pan for 5 minutes. Then, transfer the bread to a wire rack to cool completely.

7. Once cooled, slice and serve the Sussex Soy Bread.

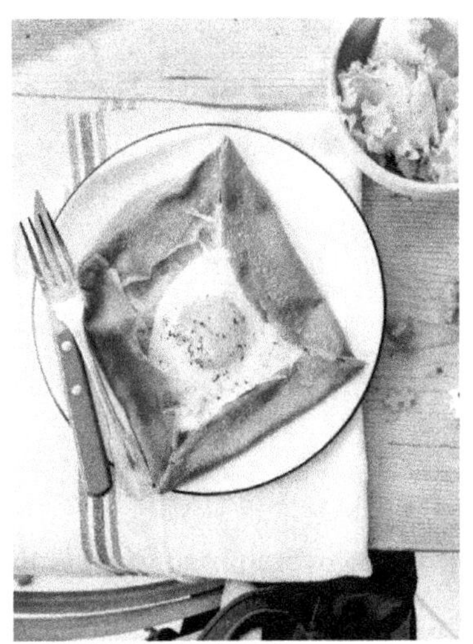

Soy and Buckwheat Crepes

Prep Time	Cook Time	Servings
10 min	15 min	4

INGREDIENTS:

- 3 eggs
- ⅓ cup heaped buckwheat flour
- ½ cup heaped soy flour
- ½ tsp cinnamon
- ¼ tsp ground nutmeg
- 1 beaten egg
- 1 ¼ cups unsweetened soy milk
- 2 tbsp soy oil

Method:

8. Buckwheat flour and soy flour into a large mixing bowl. Add the cinnamon and ground nutmeg to the bowl and create a well in the center. Pour the beaten egg into the well and slowly mix it with a wooden spoon. Gradually pour the soy milk while beating the mixture, creating a smooth batter. Cover the bowl and let the batter

For Serving:

- Stewed fruit or sugar-free jam

Nutritional Value:

- Calories: 384
- Calories: 341
- Carbohydrates: 21.8 g
- Protein: 19.4 g
- Fat: 17.6 g

stand in the refrigerator for 10-30 minutes.

9. Heat a large non-stick frying pan over medium heat until hot. Add half of the soy oil and tilt the pan to ensure the bottom is fully coated with oil. Spoon 2 tablespoons of the batter into the pan and tilt it to spread the mixture evenly over the bottom. Cook for approximately 2 minutes or until the underside is slightly golden. Flip the crêpe over with a spatula and cook for another minute until the other half is slightly golden. Take out the cooked crêpe to a plate.

10. Repeat the process with the remaining batter and soy oil, keeping the cooked crêpes warm. Serve the crêpes warm with stewed fruit or sugar-free jam

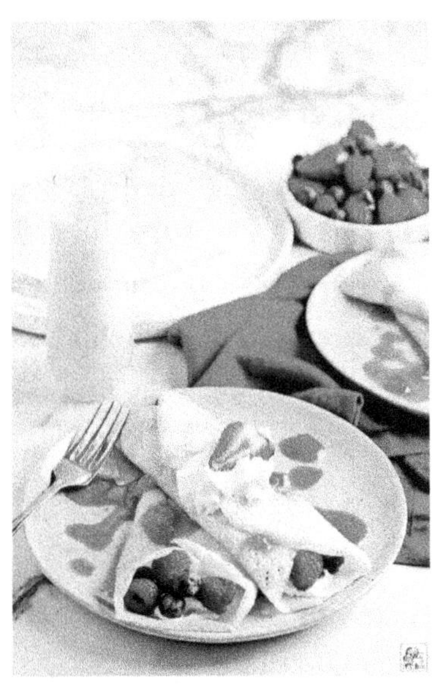

Soy and Buckwheat Crepes

Prep Time	Cook Time	Servings
10 min	15 min	4

INGREDIENTS:

- ½ cup heaped soy flour
- ¼ cup rice flour
- 1 beaten egg
- 1 ¼ cups

unsweetened soy milk

- 2 tbsp soy oil

Method:

1. Sift the soy and rice flour into a large mixing bowl, creating a well in the center. Add the beaten egg into the well and beat slowly with a wooden spoon to mix everything. Pour in the soy milk and continue beating until a smooth batter forms. Cover the batter and let it stand in the refrigerator for 10-30 minutes.

2. Heat a large non-stick frying pan over medium heat until hot. Add

For Serving:

- Berries with honey

or sugar-free jam

Nutritional Value:

- Calories: 328

- Carbohydrates: 19.1 g

- Protein: 19 g

- Fat: 18.4 g

half of the soy oil to the pan and tilt it to ensure the bottom is coated with oil. Spoon 2 tablespoons of the batter into the pan and tilt it to spread the mixture evenly across the bottom. Wait for approximately two minutes or until tiny bubbles start forming on the surface. When the crêpe is slightly golden. Use a spatula to flip the crêpe over and cook for another minute or until the other side is slightly golden. Transfer the cooked crêpe to a plate.

3. Repeat the process with the remaining batter and soy oil, keeping the cooked crêpes warm. Serve the crêpes warm with berries, drizzle honey, or top with sugar-free jam.

4.

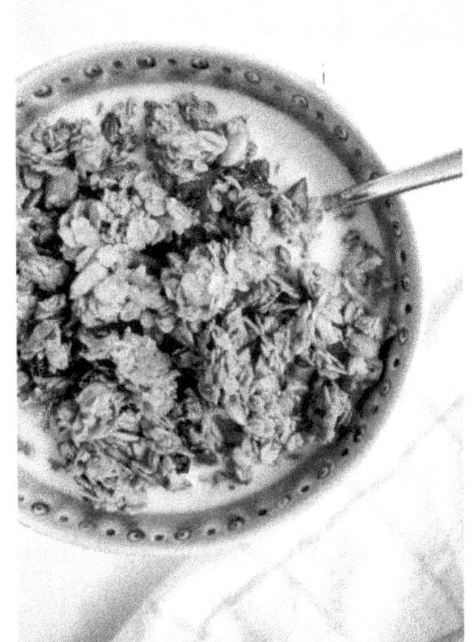

Crunchy Almond Granola

Prep Time	Cook Time	Servings
10 min	35 min	10

INGREDIENTS:

- 4 ½ cups rolled oats
- ⅔ cup sunflower seeds
- 1 ⅔ cups chopped almonds
- ⅔ cup brown rice malt
- ⅔ cup soy oil
- ⅔ cup apple juice
- 2 cups raisins
- 1 cup

desiccated/dried

shredded heaped coconut

Method:

1. Preheat the oven to 150°C/300°F/Gas 2. Combine the rolled oats, sunflower seeds, and chopped almonds in a large mixing bowl.

2. Whisk together the brown rice malt, soy oil, and apple juice in a separate jug. Pour this mixture over the dry ingredients in the bowl and mix well.

3. Spread the mixture evenly onto a baking sheet and bake for approximately 35 minutes or until

For Serving:

- Soy milk or soy yogurt

Nutritional Value:

- Calories: 428

- Carbohydrates: 31.1 g

- Protein: 10 g

- Fat: 29 g

it turns light brown. Stir the mixture every 5-10 minutes during baking to ensure even toasting.

4. Remove the baking sheet from the oven and allow the granola to cool. Once cooled, transfer it back to the mixing bowl.

5. Stir in the raisins and desiccated/dried shredded coconut, ensuring they are evenly distributed throughout the granola.

6. Serve the crunchy almond granola with soy milk or soy yogurt. The remaining granola can be stored in an airtight container for up to 4 weeks.

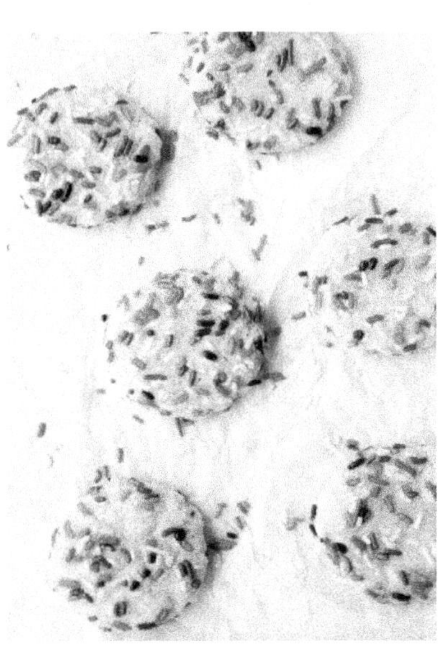

INGREDIENTS:

- ½ cup pumpkin seeds
- ⅓ cup golden flaxseeds
- ⅓ cup heaped almonds
- ½ cup sunflower seeds

Nutritional Value:

- Calories: 240
- Carbohydrates: 8.7 g
- Protein: 9.3 g
- Fat: 12 g

Phyto Sprinkle

Prep Time	Cook Time	Servings
5 min	None	8

Method:

1. Place all the ingredients in a blender or food processor.

2. Pulse the ingredients briefly until they are coarsely chopped.

3. Sprinkle the mixture over cereal or fruit and yogurt when serving.

4. Store the remaining Phyto Sprinkle in an airtight container for up to 4 weeks.

For Serving:

- Cereal Fruit

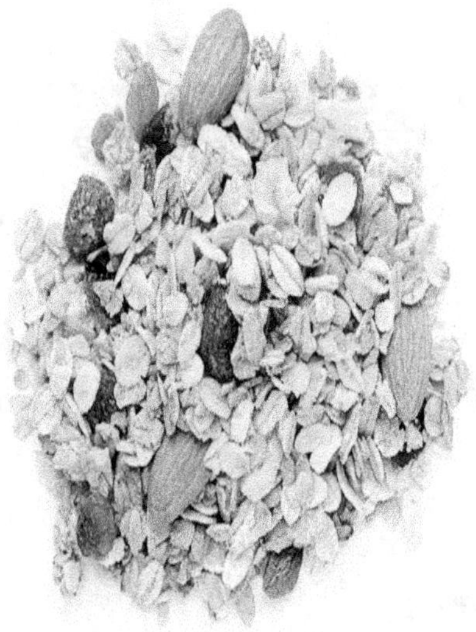

Phyto Muesli

Prep Time	Cook Time	Servings
5 min	None	10

INGREDIENTS:

- 4 ½ cups rolled oats
- 1 ¼ cups puffed rice
- 8 cups cornflakes
- ⅔ cup chopped almonds
- ½ cup pumpkin seeds
- ¾ cup heaped chopped

pecans

- ⅔ cup sesame seeds
- ⅔ cup pine nuts

Method:

1. In a large mixing bowl, combine all the ingredients.

2. Mix them until well combined.

3. Serve the Phyto Muesli with soy yogurt or soy milk and fruit.

4. The remaining muesli can be stored in an airtight container for up to 4 weeks.

- ½ cup heaped flaxseeds
- 1 cup heaped raisins
- ½ cup heaped unsulphured dried chopped apricots

For Serving:

- Soy milk or soy yogurt
- Fruit

Nutritional Value:

- Calories: 451

- Carbohydrates: 44.1 g

- Protein: 12.8 g

- Fat: 25 g

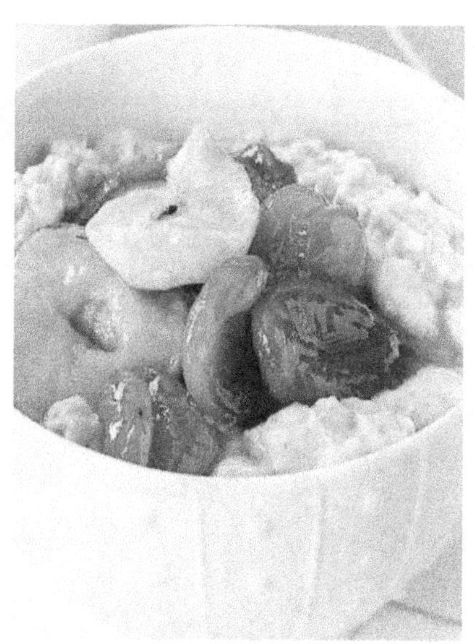

Porridge with Spiced Fruit Compote

Prep Time	Cook Time	Servings
5 min	20 min	4

INGREDIENTS:

- 1 ¾ cups rolled oats
- 4 cups soy milk
- Salt

Compote:

- ½ cup scant

caster/superfine sugar

- 1 cup scant dried figs,

chopped

- ½ cup unsulphured
- heaped dried apricots,

chopped

Method:

1. To make the compote, pour 1 cup of water into a medium-sized saucepan. Add the sugar, dried fruit, cinnamon sticks, cloves, and lemon zest. Heat the mixture over medium heat until it reaches boiling point, then lower the heat to a gentle level and let it simmer for approximately 10 minutes, or until the fruit becomes tender and plump, and the liquid has dissipated.

102

- 3 tbsp dried cranberries
- 2 cinnamon sticks
- 4 cloves
- Juice of 1 lemon, plus

2 strips of zest

For Serving:

- Plain yogurt or serving

Nutritional Value:

- Calories: 442

- Carbohydrates: 77.9 g

- Protein: 15.2 g

- Fat: 8 g

-

2. Add the lemon juice to the pan. Remove the pan from the heat and set it aside for 2 minutes to cool slightly.

3. In a medium-sized saucepan, combine the oats and soy milk. Season lightly with salt. Bring to a boil, then reduce the heat to low and let it simmer for about 10 minutes, stirring continuously, until the porridge is thick and creamy.

4. Serve the hot porridge with the fruit compote and yogurt.

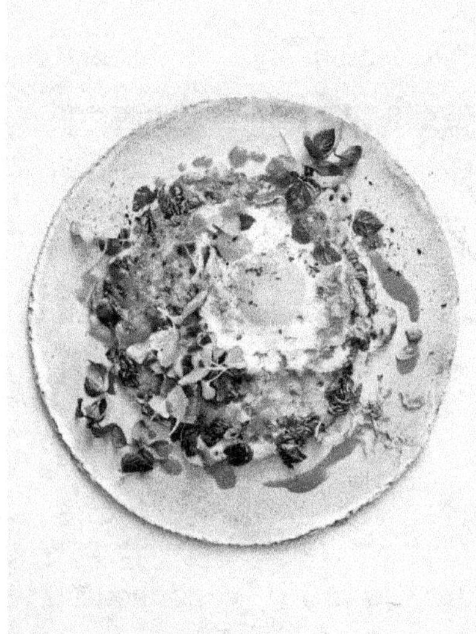

Chili & Corn Fritters With Scrambled Eggs

Prep Time	Cook Time	Servings
20 min	20 min	4

INGREDIENTS:

- 1 ¼ cups plain/ all-purpose flour
- 1 tsp baking powder
- 2 eggs, beaten
- ½ cup unsweetened soy milk
- 1 cup canned drained
- and rinsed sweetcorn/ corn kernels
- 1 small finely chopped red chili

Method:

1. To make the compote, pour 1 cup of water into a medium-sized saucepan. Add the sugar, dried Sift the flour and baking powder into a large mixing bowl. Make a well in the middle and add the beaten eggs. Slowly beat the eggs with a wooden spoon to mix them. Pour in the soy milk and add the sweetcorn/corn kernels and chopped chili. Season lightly with salt and pepper. Beat the mixture

104

- 2 tbsp vegetable oil
- 8 baby halved plum

tomatoes

- 6 slices of prosciutto
- Salt and freshly ground

black pepper

For Serving:

- Baby spinach leaves

Nutritional Value:

- Calories: 226
- Carbohydrates: 15.7 g
- Protein: 13.5 g
- Fat: 12 g

Scrambled eggs:

- 4 eggs
- ¼ cup unsweetened soy
- Milk 30g/1oz/2 tbsp butter
- Freshly ground black pepper

-

until a smooth batter forms. Cover the batter and let it stand in the refrigerator for 10-30 minutes.

2. Heat a large non-stick frying pan over medium heat until hot. Add half the vegetable oil and tilt the pan to ensure the bottom is completely coated. Spoon 2 tablespoons of the batter into the pan and cook for 2 minutes or until golden brown. Flip the cake over with a spatula and cook for another 2 minutes or until golden brown and cooked through. Remove the cake from the pan, drain it on kitchen paper, and keep it warm. Repeat the process with the remaining batter and oil.

3. Meanwhile, preheat the grill/broiler to medium. Grill/broil the halved baby plum tomatoes and prosciutto slices for 2 minutes or until the prosciutto turns slightly golden.

4. For the scrambled eggs, beat the eggs in a small mixing bowl. Stir in the soy milk and season lightly with black pepper. Melt the butter in a non-stick frying pan over low heat. Pour in the egg mixture and cook gently, stirring frequently, for a few minutes until the eggs are set.

5. Serve the warm cakes topped with grilled/broiled prosciutto and tomatoes. Accompany the cakes with scrambled eggs on a bed of baby spinach leaves.

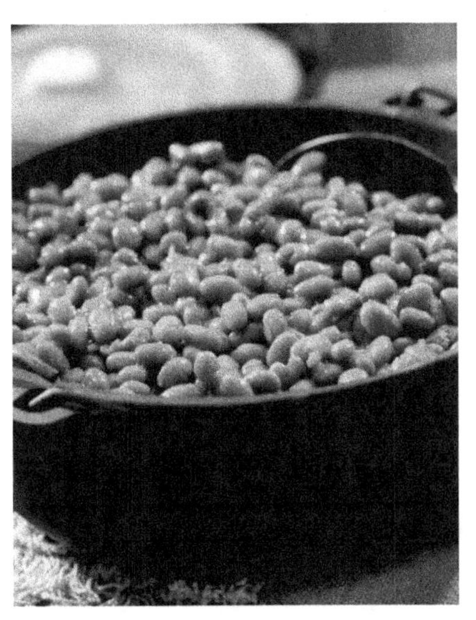

Crunchy Almond
Granola

Prep Time	Cook Time	Servings
10 min	20 min	1

Method:

INGREDIENTS:

- 4 ½ cups rolled oats
- Extra virgin olive oil
- 1 tbsp tomato puree
- ½ tsp smoked paprika
- 1 ½ cups passata
- 1 tsp coconut sugar
- 1 tsp tamari soy sauce
- Handful of spinach

leaves (optional)

1. In a saucepan, heat a tablespoon of olive oil over medium heat. Add the chopped onion and garlic and sauté until softened.

2. Stir in the tomato puree, smoked paprika, finely chopped sage leaves, coconut sugar, and tamari soy sauce. Allow the mixture to simmer for a few minutes.

3. Add the cannellini beans and passata to the saucepan. Continue

- Sea salt and ground

black pepper

- ½ onion, finely chopped
- 1 garlic clove, finely

chopped

- ½ tsp fresh sage leaves,

finely

chopped

- 3 ¼ cups canned

cannellini

beans, rinsed and drained

Nutritional Value:

- Calories: 257
- Carbohydrates: 35.1 g
- Protein: 5.6 g
- Fat: 10.5 g
-

simmering until the liquid around the beans has reduced and thickened. Season with sea salt and freshly ground black pepper to taste.

4. Add a handful of spinach leaves to the beans and stir until wilted.

5. Serve the homemade baked beans as a delicious and healthy breakfast option.

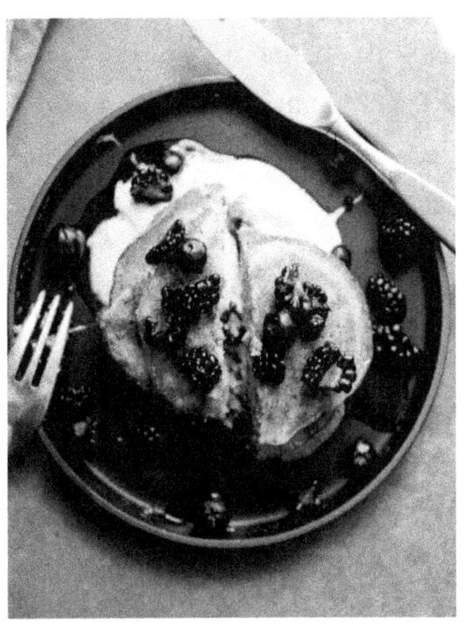

Almond and Coconut Pancake

Prep Time	Cook Time	Servings
5 min	10 min	2

Method:

INGREDIENTS:

- Coconut oil for cooking
- 2 eggs
- 4 tbsp sparkling water
- 2 tbsp ground almonds
- 2 tbsp coconut flour
- Pinch of salt

1. In a saucepan, heat a tablespoon of olive oil over medium heat. Add the chopped onion and garlic and sauté until softened.

2. Mix the ground almonds, coconut flour, eggs, sparkling water, and a pinch of salt in a bowl. Stir until the mixture is smooth and there are no lumps.

3. Heat a teaspoon of coconut oil in a frying pan over medium heat.

109

Nutritional Value:

- Calories: 327

- Carbohydrates: 3.5 g

- Protein: 11.2 g

- Fat: 29 g

4. Use a 1/4 cup measure to spoon the pancake batter into the pan. Look for bubbling or browning of the edges before flipping the pancake.

5. Cook the pancakes on both sides until they are golden brown.

6. Serve the almond and coconut pancakes with toppings of your choice, such as fresh fruit, yogurt, or maple syrup.

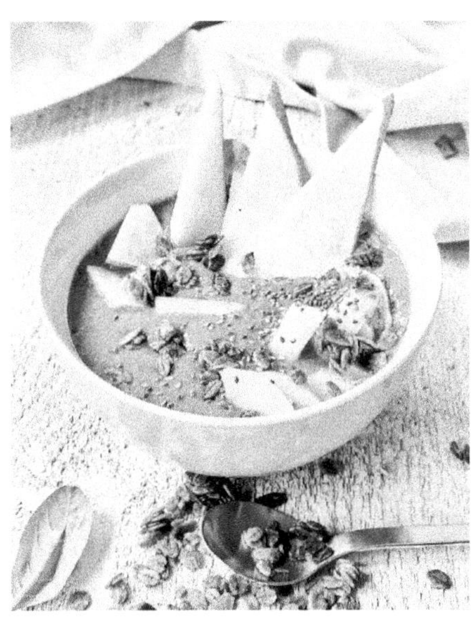

Green Smoothie Bowl

Prep Time	Cook Time	Servings
5 min	None	2

INGREDIENTS:

- Handful of kale or spinach

- 1 banana (frozen)

- ½ ripe avocado

- 1 cup unsweetened soya, coconut, or almond milk

Method:

1. Combine the frozen banana, ripe avocado, a handful of spinach or kale, and unsweetened soya, coconut, or almond milk in a blender.

2. Blend the ingredients quickly until the mixture is completely smooth and creamy.

3. Pour the green smoothie into a bowl.

111

Nutritional Value:

- Calories: 180

- Carbohydrates: 13.7 g

- Protein: 6.5 g

- Fat: 11.2 g

4. Garnish the smoothie bowl with the toppings of your preference, such as slices of fresh fruit, berries, shredded coconut, or a drizzle of nut butter. Feel at liberty to exercise your creativity and add your favorite toppings.

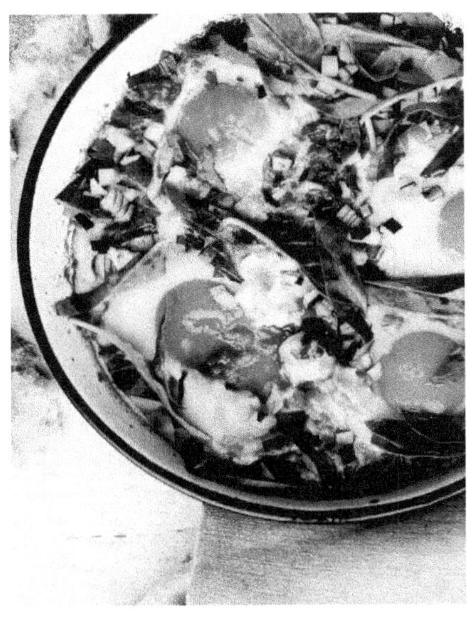

Berber Eggs

Prep Time   Cook Time   Servings

5 min   15 min   2

Method:

INGREDIENTS:

- 4 eggs
- 1 red onion, finely

chopped

- ½ red chili, finely

chopped

- 2 garlic cloves, crushed
- 14 oz can chopped

tomatoes

1. Heat a frying pan over medium heat and add a little oil. Sauté the finely chopped red onion, red chili, and crushed garlic for a few minutes until softened.

2. Add the chopped tomatoes, halved cherry tomatoes, smoked paprika, and a little water to the pan. Cook the mixture for about five minutes, allowing the flavors to blend.

3. Crack the eggs into the tomato sauce, spacing them out evenly. Cover the pan with a lid and cook

113

- 1 cup cherry tomatoes, halved

- ½ tsp smoked paprika
- 2 tbsp fresh coriander

Nutritional Value:

- Calories: 210
- Carbohydrates: 10 g
- Protein: 17.6 g
- Fat: 10.2 g

for approximately eight minutes until the egg whites are set and the yolks are still slightly runny.

4. Scatter fresh coriander over the cooked eggs.

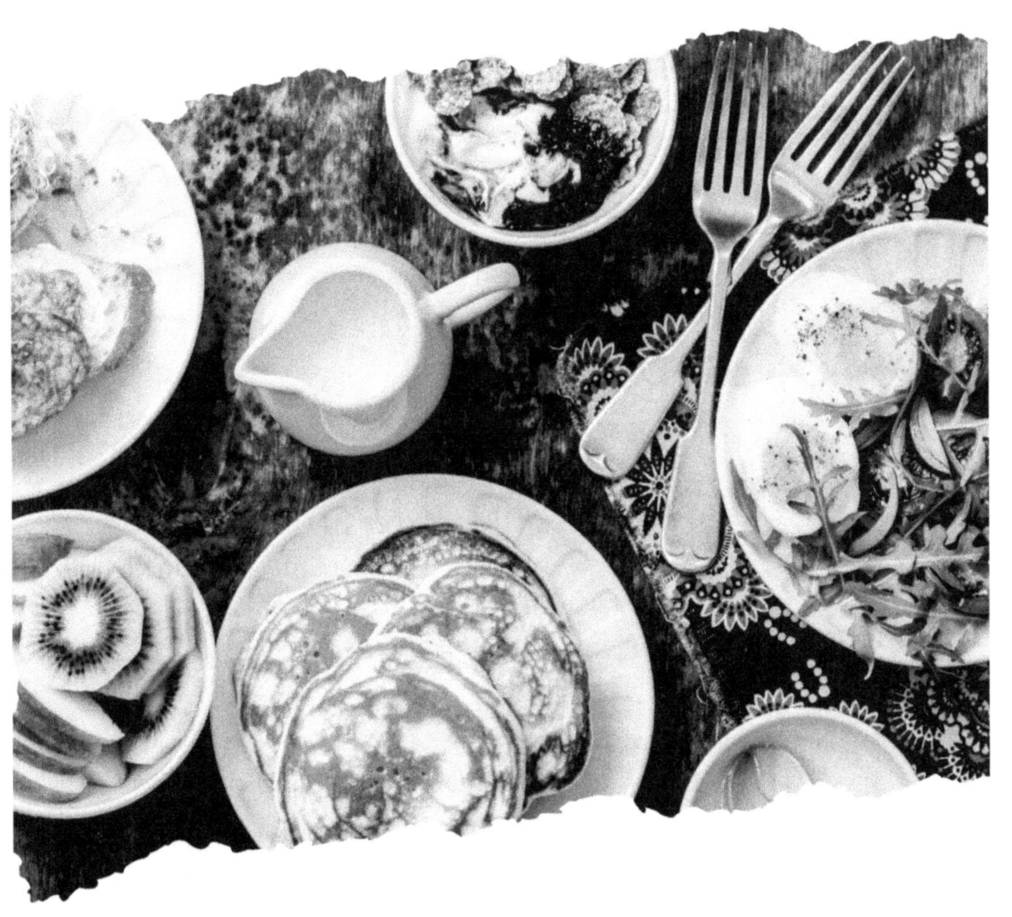

Lunch Recipes

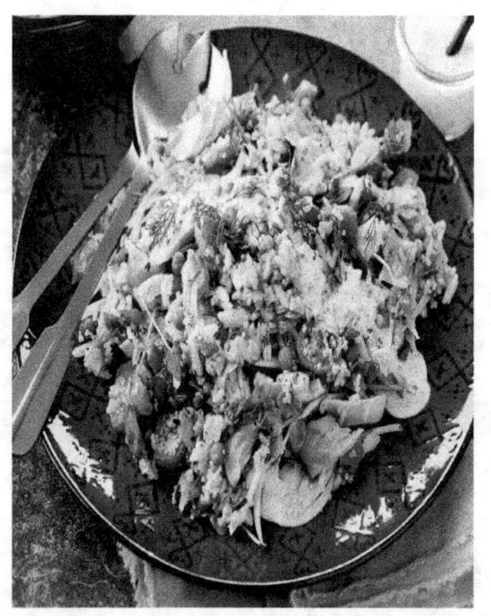

Brown Rice & Watercress Salad

Prep Time	Cook Time	Servings
5 min	25 min	3

Method:

1. Heat a frying pan over medium heat and add a little oil. Sauté the finely chopped red onion, red chili, and crushed garlic for a few minutes until softened.

2. Combine the brown rice with 2 cups of cold water in a saucepan. Bring to a boil over high heat, then reduce the heat to medium, and let it simmer for 25 minutes or until the rice is tender and the water has been absorbed. Transfer the

INGREDIENTS:

- 4 eggs
- 1 cup scant long-grain brown rice
- 1 bunch watercress, roughly chopped
- ½ cup canned, drained & rinsed sweetcorn/corn kernels

116

- 1 green pepper,

deseeded and chopped

- Freshly ground black

Pepper

For serving:

- Salad dressing

Nutritional Value:

- Calories: 353
- Carbohydrates: 73.1 g
- Protein: 8 g
- Fat: 3.4 g
-

cooked rice to a serving bowl and allow it to cool.

3. Add the roughly chopped watercress, canned sweetcorn, and green pepper to the serving bowl with the cooled rice. Season with freshly ground black pepper.

4. Mix all the ingredients until well combined.

5. Serve the Brown Rice & Watercress Salad with your choice of salad dressing.

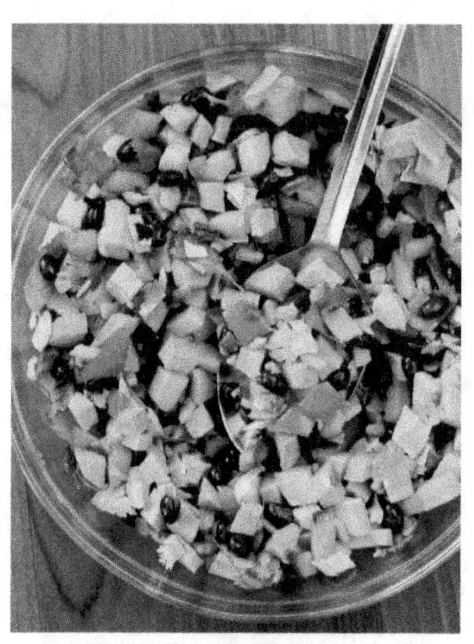

Sweet Potato Salad

Prep Time	Cook Time	Servings
10 min	10 min	3

INGREDIENTS:

- 2 spring onions, chopped

- 1 tbsp parsley leaves, chopped

- 1 tbsp basil leaves, chopped
- 3 ½ cups sweet potatoes, peeled and cubed

- 1-2 garlic cloves, crushed

Method:

1. Place the peeled and cubed sweet potatoes in a steamer and steam them over high heat for approximately 10 minutes or until tender. Transfer the steamed sweet potatoes to a serving bowl and allow them to cool.

2. Add the crushed garlic cloves, chopped parsley leaves, chopped basil leaves, chopped chives, chopped spring onions, soy oil, and the juice of one lemon to the

- 1 green pepper,
- 1 tbsp chives, chopped
- 1 tbsp soy oil
- Juice of 1 lemon
- Freshly ground

black pepper

Nutritional Value:

- Calories: 273
- Carbohydrates: 52 g
- Protein: 3.4 g
- Fat: 5.8 g

serving bowl with the sweet potatoes. Season with freshly ground black pepper.

3. Mix all the ingredients until well combined.

4. Serve the Sweet Potato Salad.

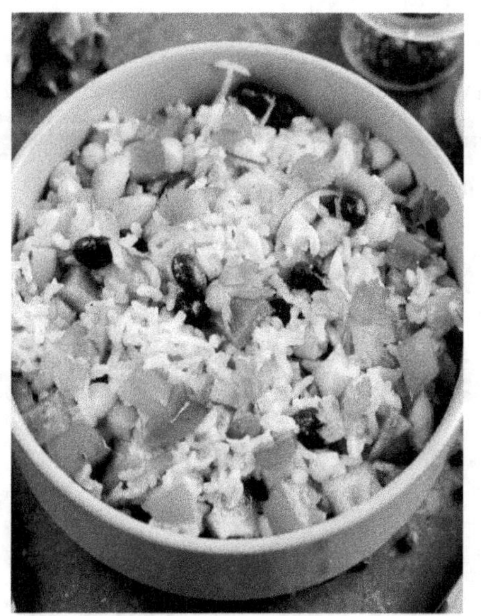

Oriental Rice Salad

Prep Time	Cook Time	Servings
10 min	20 min	4

INGREDIENTS:

- 2 spring onions,
- ¼ cup long-grain

white or brown rice

- ¾ cup basmati rice
- 1 tbsp sunflower oil
- 6 spring onions/scallions

finely chopped

- 1 red pepper, deseeded

and thinly sliced lengthways

Method:

1. In a saucepan, cook both types of rice in boiling water over medium heat for 12-15 minutes or until tender. Drain the rice, rinse it with boiling water, and drain again. Set it aside.

2. Heat sunflower oil in a frying pan over medium heat. Add the finely chopped spring onions/scallions, red pepper slices, yellow pepper slices, mangetout/snow peas, and bean sprouts. Fry the vegetables

120

- 1 green pepper,
- 1 deseeded & thinly

sliced yellow pepper

- ½ cup mangetout/

snow peas

- 1 cup heaped bean sprouts
- 2 tbsp tamari or soy sauce
- 1 tbsp lemon juice
- ⅓ cup sprouted mung

beans heaped

- Freshly ground black

pepper

Nutritional Value:

- Calories: 256
- Carbohydrates: 46.7 g
- Protein: 8.3 g
- Fat: 4.5 g

for a few minutes, occasionally stirring, until they become tender and lightly browned.

3. Add tamari or soy sauce, lemon juice, sprouted mung beans, and cooked rice to the frying pan. Season the mixture with freshly ground black pepper. Stir continuously, ensuring that all the grains are evenly coated with the sauce.

5. Serve the Oriental Rice Salad, either hot or cold

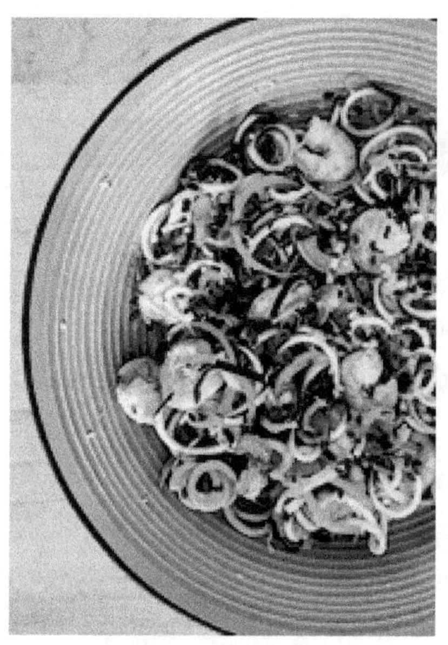

Summer Salad

Prep Time	Cook Time	Servings
10 min	5 min	2

INGREDIENTS:

- 4 carrots, peeled, cut into ribbons
- 4 baby turnips, peeled, cut into ribbons
- 1 ¼ cups shelled broad/fava beans
- 2 courgettes/zucchini, cut into ribbons
- ½ cup baby spinach
- Freshly ground black pepper

Method:

1. Place the shelled broad/fava beans in a steamer and steam them over high heat for approximately 5 minutes or until lightly cooked. Transfer the steamed broad beans to a serving bowl and allow them to cool completely.

2. Add the courgette/zucchini ribbons, carrot ribbons, baby turnip ribbons, and baby spinach to the serving bowl with the cooled

For serving:

- Salad dressing

Nutritional Value:

- Calories: 92
- Carbohydrates: 17.1 g
- Protein: 5.4 g
- Fat: 0.2 g
-

broad beans. Mix all the ingredients until well combined.

3. Season the salad with freshly ground black pepper.

4. Serve the Summer Salad with your choice of salad dressing.

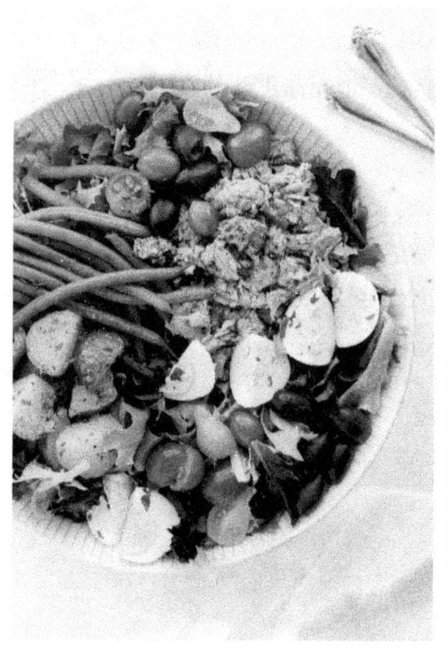

Nicoise Salad with Soy Dressing

Prep Time	Cook Time	Servings
20 min	2 5 min	4

INGREDIENTS:

- 2 cups fine/thin green beans
- 10 cherry tomatoes, halved
- 3 eggs
- 8 small potatoes, halved
- 4 tuna steaks
- Olive oil for brushing
- ¾ cup black olives
- 1 roughly torn leaves baby cos/romaine lettuce

Method:

1. Place the eggs in a small saucepan and cover them with cold water. Bring to a boil over high heat, then reduce the heat to low, and let it simmer for 5 minutes. Remove the pan from the heat, drain the water, and rinse the eggs under cold running water for 1 minute. Leave the eggs in the pan of cold water for an additional 2 minutes, then peel and set them aside.

124

Dressing:

- Salad dressing
- 1 tsp Dijon mustard
- 2 tbsp lime juice
- 1 garlic clove, chopped
- 1 ½ cups silken tofu
- ½ cup scant unsweetened

soy milk

- Freshly ground

black pepper

Nutritional Value:

- Calories: 650
- Carbohydrates: 49 g
- Protein: 48.7 g
- Fat: 28.5 g

2. Cook the potatoes in a saucepan of boiling water over high heat for approximately 10 minutes or until tender. Drain the potatoes and let them cool.

3. Preheat the grill/broiler to high. Lightly brush the tuna steaks with olive oil and grill/broil them on each side for 2-3 minutes until browned on the outside and slightly pink in the middle. Use a fork to break the tuna into bite-size pieces.

4. Steam the green beans for about 5 minutes. Remove the steamer from the heat, rinse the beans under cold running water, drain well, and transfer them to a large salad bowl.

5. Cut the boiled eggs in half and add them to the bowl with the beans. Add the cooked potatoes, grilled tuna, cherry tomatoes, black

olives, and torn lettuce leaves. Gently toss all the ingredients together.

6. To make the dressing, combine the silken tofu, unsweetened soy milk, chopped garlic clove, Dijon mustard, lime juice, and freshly ground black pepper in a blender or food processor. Blend until smooth. Season lightly with additional black pepper if desired.

7. Drizzle the soy dressing over the salad and serve.

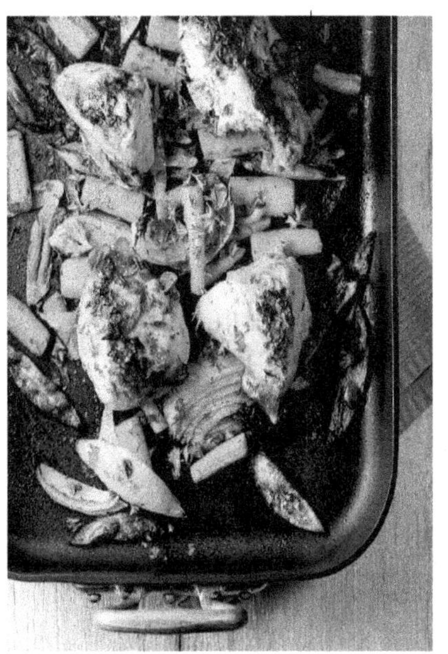

Roasted Dijon Chicken

Prep Time   Cook Time   Servings

5 min   1hr.30 min   6

INGREDIENTS:

- 2 tbsp olive oil
- 2 tbsp Dijon mustard
- 1 quartered lemon
- 1 garlic bulb, sliced

at the top

- 1 whole chicken

(approximately 1.5 kg)

Method:

1. . Preheat the oven to 400°F/Gas

2. In a small bowl, combine the olive oil and Dijon mustard.

3. Place the whole chicken in an ovenproof dish and coat it with the olive oil and mustard mixture.

4. Stuff the chicken cavity with the lemon quarters.

5. Cook the chicken in the oven for 20 minutes.

127

For serving:

- Roasted root vegetables

(carrots, sweet potatoes,

parsnips)

Nutritional Value:

- Calories: 92
- Calories: 327
- Carbohydrates: 0.8 g
- Protein: 48.9 g
- Fat: 14.2 g

6. Flip the chicken over and add the sliced garlic to the dish. Peel and chop the root vegetables and add them to the dish.

7. Baste the chicken with its juices and continue cooking for another 20 minutes.

8. Flip the chicken over one last time, baste it again, and cook for 20-35 minutes, or until the juices run clear and the leg joints can be easily detached with a knife and fork.

9. Remove the chicken from the oven and let it rest for 5 minutes.

5. Serve the roasted Dijon chicken with the roasted root vegetables.

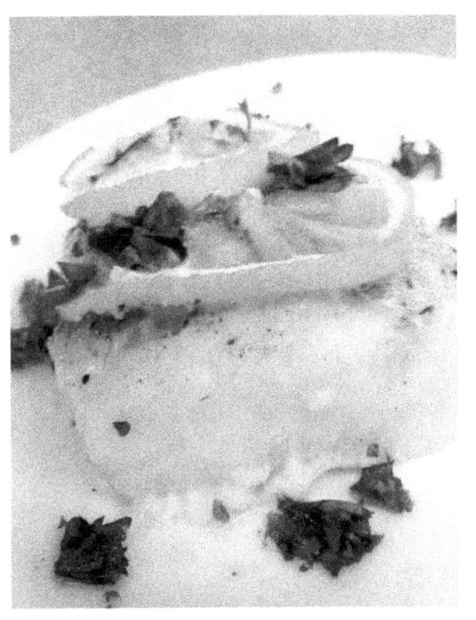

Baked Cod with Lemon Sauce

Prep Time	Cook Time	Servings
5 min	1hr.15 min	4

INGREDIENTS:

- 4 5-oz cod fillets
- ½ cup butter or ghee
- 1 cup crème fraiche
- 2 crushed garlic cloves
- 1 ½ tbsp Dijon mustard
- 2 tbsp lemon juice
- Sea salt & freshly

ground black pepper

Method:

1. Preheat the oven to 425°F/Gas Place the cod fillets in a baking dish, leaving some space between them. Season with sea salt and freshly ground black pepper.

2. In a small pan over low heat, melt the butter or ghee. Add the crème fraiche, crushed garlic, Dijon mustard, and lemon juice. Stir well to combine until the mixture is smooth.

129

To garnish:

- Flat-leaf parsley

For serving:

- Steamed new

potatoes

- Wilted spinach
- Lemon wedges

Nutritional Value:

- Calories: 322
- Carbohydrates:

2.6 g

- Protein: 24.4 g
- Fat: 24.5 g

3. Pour the lemon sauce over the cod fillets into the baking dish.

4. Bake the cod in the oven for 10-15 minutes or until the fish is cooked and flakes easily with a knife.

5. Serve the baked cod immediately with steamed new potatoes, wilted spinach, and lemon wedges. Garnish with flat-leaf parsley.

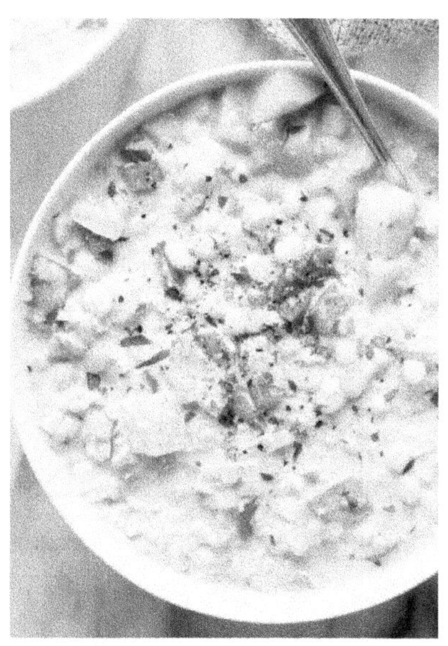

INGREDIENTS:

- 1 potato, diced
- 1 celery stalk, diced
- 1 vegetable stock cube
- 2 tbsp olive oil
- 1 small onion, finely

chopped

- 3 garlic cloves, finely

chopped

Corn Chowder with Garlic Prawns

Prep Time	Cook Time	Servings
15 min	20 min	4

Method:

1. Heat 1 tablespoon of olive oil in a saucepan over medium heat. Add the finely chopped onion and 1/3 of the finely chopped garlic. Cook for 3 minutes, stirring occasionally, until the onion is translucent. Add the diced potato and cook for another 2 minutes until the potatoes are heated.

2. Stir in the sweetcorn, diced celery, and unsweetened soy milk. Season with freshly ground black pepper. Crumble in the vegetable stock

- 3 cups unsweetened soy milk

- 2 cups peeled uncooked prawns/shrimp

- 4 handfuls flat-leaf parsley leaves, chopped

- Freshly ground black pepper

- 1 cup canned drained and rinsed sweetcorn/ corn kernels

Nutritional Value:

- Calories: 319

- Carbohydrates: 42.7 g

- Protein: 23.7 g

- Fat: 5.9 g

cube. Cover the saucepan with a lid and bring the mixture to a boil over high heat. Reduce the heat to low. Let it simmer for 10 minutes or until the vegetables are tender.

3. Heat the remaining tablespoon of olive oil over medium-high heat in a separate frying pan. Add the remaining finely chopped garlic and the peeled, uncooked prawns/shrimp. Fry, stirring frequently, for about 2 minutes or until the prawns/shrimp turn pink.

4. Remove the frying pan from heat, add the chopped flat-leaf parsley, and stir thoroughly.

5. Spoon the corn chowder into bowls and top with the garlic prawns/shrimp.

6. Serve the Corn Chowder with Garlic Prawns immediately.

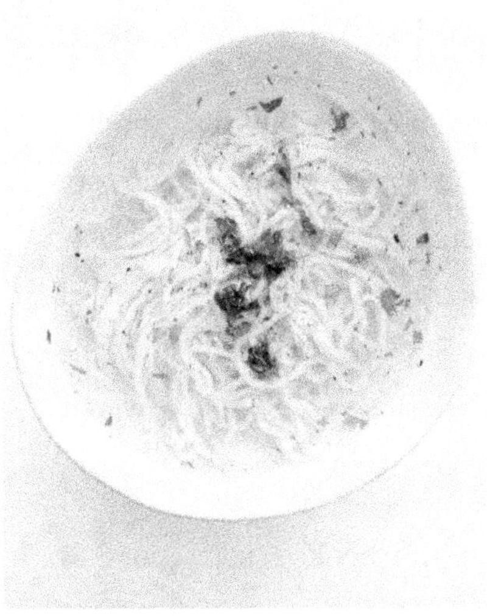

Chicken Noodle Soup

Prep Time	Cook Time	Servings
15 min	20 min	4

INGREDIENTS:

- 2 cups soba noodles
- 4 cups chicken stock
- 1 garlic clove, finely chopped
- 2 lemongrass sticks, finely chopped
- 1-inch piece peeled and grated root ginger
- 2 skinless, cut into strips
- boneless chicken breasts

Method:

1. Pour the chicken stock into a large saucepan. Add the finely chopped garlic, grated ginger, and chopped lemongrass. Cover the saucepan with a lid and bring the mixture to a boil over medium heat. Reduce the heat to low, add the chicken strips, and let it simmer for 8-10 minutes or until the chicken is cooked.

2. Add the shiitake mushrooms and broccoli to the simmering soup.

133

Simmer for another 6 minutes or until the broccoli is lightly cooked.

3. Meanwhile, cook the soba noodles in a separate large saucepan according to the package instructions until they are al dente. Stir occasionally. Drain the noodles, rinse with boiling water, and drain again.

4. Divide the cooked soba noodles into serving bowls. Ladle the chicken and vegetable soup over the noodles.

5. Serve the Chicken Noodle Soup hot.

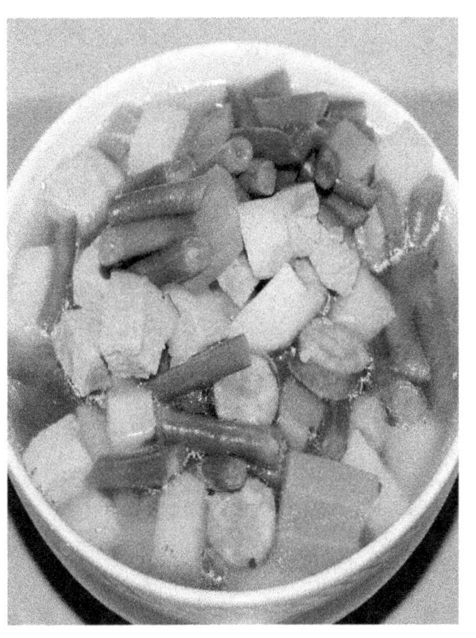

Edamame Bean & Vegetable Soup

Prep Time	Cook Time	Servings
10 min	20 min	4

INGREDIENTS:

- 4 cups vegetable stock
- 2 large carrots, grated
- 2 finely sliced leeks
- 1 small handful thyme,

chopped

- 1 3/4 drained and

rinsed (canned or

frozen) Edamame beans

Method:

6. Pour the chicken stock into a large saucepan. Add the finely chopped garlic, grated ginger, and chopped

7. Rinse the edamame beans thoroughly and drain. Place them in a saucepan and pour in the vegetable stock. Bring to a boil over high heat, then reduce the heat to low, cover with a lid, and let it simmer for about 5 minutes or until the beans are tender.

135

- 1 large parsnip, peeled

- and grated

- Freshly ground black

pepper

Nutritional Value:

- Calories: 96

- Carbohydrates: 15.7 g

- Protein: 5.2 g

- Fat: 1.5 g

8. Transfer the mixture to a blender or food processor and blend until smooth. Pour the blended mixture back into the saucepan.

9. Add the grated carrots, parsnip, and sliced leeks to the saucepan. Simmer for 10 minutes to cook the vegetables.

10. Stir in the chopped thyme and let it simmer for an additional 5 minutes. Season with freshly ground black pepper.

11. Serve the Edamame Bean & Vegetable Soup hot.

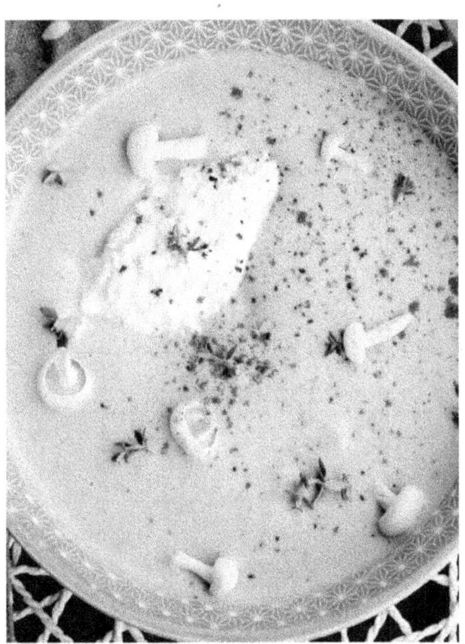

Mushroom & Mint Soup

Prep Time	Cook Time	Servings
10 min	45 min	4

INGREDIENTS:

- 4 large potatoes, chopped
- 1 small onion, chopped
- 4 cups scant chicken stock
- 1 ¾ oz soy margarine
- 8 oz mushrooms, sliced
- 1 tbsp plain/all-purpose flour
- 2 tbsp finely chopped mint leaves

Method:

1. Combine the chopped potatoes, onion, chicken stock, lemon juice, zest, and chopped rosemary in a large saucepan. Season with freshly ground black pepper. Cover with a lid and bring to a boil over high heat. Reduce the heat to low, and let it simmer for 25 minutes, stirring occasionally, or until the vegetables are tender. Allow the mixture to cool for 10 minutes.

137

- ⅔ cup scant unsweetened soy milk

- Juice and zest of 1 lemon
- 1 tbsp chopped rosemary leaves

- Freshly ground black pepper

Nutritional Value:

- Calories: 381

- Carbohydrates: 60.5 g

- Protein: 13.5 g

- Fat: 9.5 g

2. Transfer the cooked vegetables to a blender or food processor and blend until smooth.

3. In a small saucepan, melt the soy margarine over low heat. Add the sliced mushrooms and stir until they are coated in the margarine. Cook for about 10 minutes, stirring occasionally, until the mushrooms are dark in color. Sprinkle the flour over the mushrooms, stir gently to coat them, and set aside.

4. Return the blended soup to the saucepan and add the cooked mushrooms. Increase the heat to medium and bring the soup to a boil, stirring occasionally. Reduce the heat to low and stir in the chopped mint and soy milk. Cook for an additional 5 minutes to allow the flavors to blend.

5. Season the Mushroom & Mint
   Soup with freshly ground black
   pepper and serve.

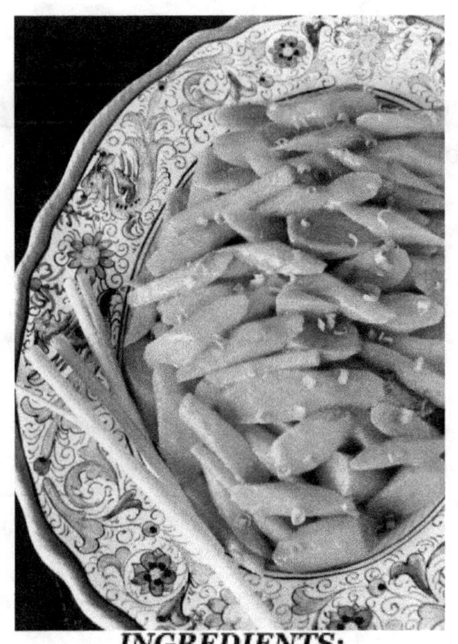

Carrot & Apricot Pâté

Prep Time	Cook Time	Servings
15 min	45 min	4

INGREDIENTS:

- Soy margarine

(for greasing)

- ¾ cup silken tofu
- ¼ cup ground almonds
- 1 tbsp lemon juice
- 1 tsp ground cardamom
- 1 tsp ground nutmeg
- 2 cups grated carrot

Method:

1. Preheat the oven to 200°C/400°F/Gas 6 and grease a small loaf pan with soy margarine. Place the finely chopped apricots in a saucepan and cover with 1/3 cup scant water. Bring to a boil over high heat, then reduce the heat to low and let it simmer for 10 minutes or until the apricots are soft.

- ½ cup finely chopped, unsulphured dried apricots

- Freshly ground black pepper

For serving:

- Green salad and toast

Nutritional Value:

- Calories: 133

- Carbohydrates: 11.8 g

- Protein: 6.1 g

- Fat: 6.9 g

2. Combine the silken tofu, ground almonds, lemon juice, ground cardamom, ground nutmeg, and grated carrot in a bowl. Mix well using a wooden spoon. Add the cooked apricots and any remaining cooking liquid, and mix thoroughly. Season with freshly ground black pepper.

3. Spoon the mixture into the greased loaf pan, cover with foil, and bake for 45 minutes or until the pâté is firm.

4. Remove the pan from the oven and allow the pâté to cool completely. Chill in the refrigerator for 30 minutes. Once chilled, remove from the pan, slice into portions, and serve with a green salad and toast.

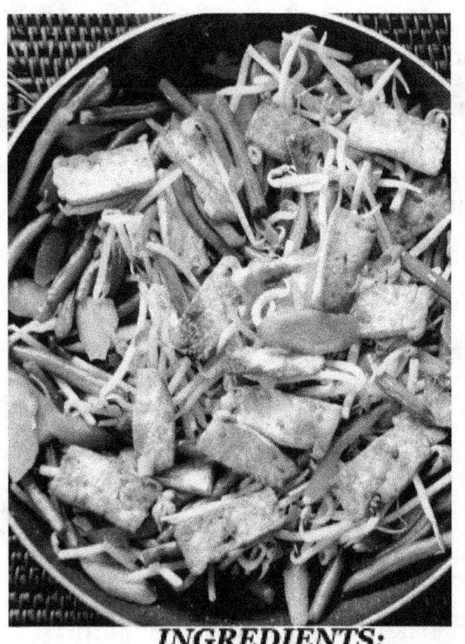

Tofu, Bean & Herb Stir- Fry

Prep Time	Cook Time	Servings
10 min	10 min	3

INGREDIENTS:

- Soy margarine
- 2 tbsp soy oil
- 2 cups cubed tofu
- 2 garlic cloves, crushed
- 2 ¼ cups green beans
- 2 tbsp tamari soy sauce

Method:

1. Heat 1 tablespoon of soy oil in a frying pan or wok over high heat until hot. Add the tofu and crushed garlic, and stir-fry for 2 minutes until the tofu absorbs the garlic flavor. Use a slotted spoon to remove the tofu and drain it on kitchen paper.

2. Heat the remaining soy oil in the same pan, then add the green beans. Stir-fry over medium heat

- ½ cup finely chopped,
- Freshly ground black

pepper

- 4 spring onions/scallions,

thinly sliced

- 3 tbsp mixed finely

chopped herbs

(such as thyme, parsley,

chives, or chervil)

For serving:

- Rice or noodles

Nutritional Value:

- Calories: 255
- Carbohydrates: 6.3 g
- Protein: 17.1 g
- Fat: 17.6 g

for about 4 minutes or until the beans are lightly cooked.

3. Add the mixed herbs, spring onions/scallions, and tamari soy sauce to the pan. Stir-fry for an additional 1 minute.

4. Return the tofu to the pan and stir-fry for 1 minute, allowing the flavors to blend. Season with freshly ground black pepper.

5. Serve the stir-fry immediately with rice or noodles.

-

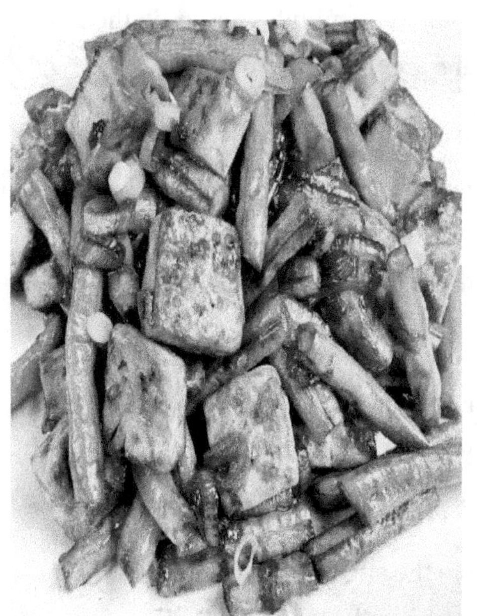

Tofu, Bean & Herb Stir-Fry

Prep Time	Cook Time	Servings
10 min	10 min	3

INGREDIENTS:

- Soy margarine
- 2 tbsp soy oil
- 2 cups cubed tofu
- 2 garlic cloves, crushed
- 2 ¼ cups green beans
- 2 tbsp tamari soy sauce

Method:

6. Heat 1 tablespoon of soy oil in a frying pan or wok over high heat until hot. Add the tofu and crushed garlic, and stir-fry for 2 minutes until the tofu absorbs the garlic flavor. Use a slotted spoon to remove the tofu and drain it on kitchen paper.

7. Heat the remaining soy oil in the same pan, then add the green

144

- ½ cup finely chopped,
- Freshly ground black

pepper

- 4 spring onions/scallions,

thinly sliced

- 3 tbsp mixed finely

chopped herbs

(such as thyme, parsley,

chives, or chervil)

For serving:

- Rice or noodles

Nutritional Value:

- Calories: 255
- Carbohydrates: 6.3 g
- Protein: 17.1 g
- Fat: 17.6 g

beans. Stir-fry over medium heat for about 4 minutes or until the beans are lightly cooked.

8. Add the mixed herbs, spring onions/scallions, and tamari soy sauce to the pan. Stir-fry for an additional 1 minute.

9. Return the tofu to the pan and stir-fry for 1 minute, allowing the flavors to blend. Season with freshly ground black pepper.

10. Serve the stir-fry immediately with rice or noodles.

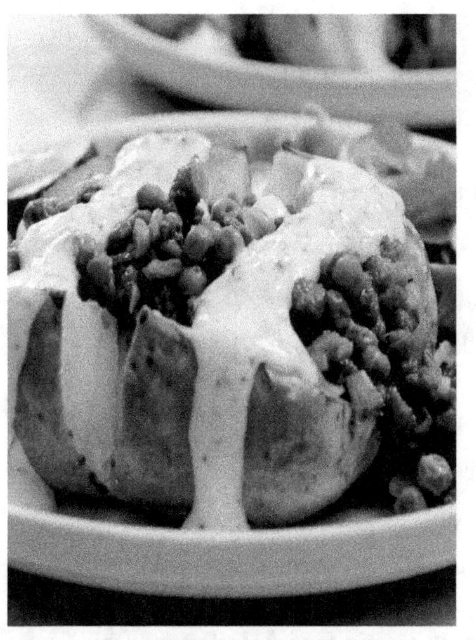

Baked Potatoes with Spicy Soybeans

Prep Time	Cook Time	Servings
15 min	3 hr min	4

INGREDIENTS:

- 2 tbsp soy oil
- 4 cups vegetable stock
- 3 bay leaves
- ¾ cup passata
- ⅔ cup molasses
- ⅔ cup Dijon mustard
- 1 large onion, chopped

Method:

1. Wash the soybeans and drain. Place them in a large bowl, cover them with cold water, and let them soak overnight or for at least 12 hours.

2. Drain the soybeans and rinse them thoroughly. Transfer them to a large saucepan, cover them with cold water, and boil over high heat. Boil for 10 minutes, then

- 2 garlic cloves, chopped
- 2 ½ cups soaked & dried

soybeans

- 4 large scrubbed

and scored baking/Idaho

potatoes

- 2 pieces of cinnamon stick
- 2 tbsp apple cider vinegar
- 1 tbsp tamari soy sauce

Nutritional Value:

- Calories: 498
- Carbohydrates: 77.8 g
- Protein: 16.7 g
- Fat: 13.6 g

reduce the heat to low. Add the bay leaves, cover with a lid, and let it simmer for 2 hours or until the soybeans are tender. Drain the soybeans and set them aside to cool.

3. Preheat the oven to 200°C/400°F/Gas 6. Place the scored potatoes on a baking tray and bake for approximately 1 hour or until tender.

4. In a saucepan, heat the soy oil over medium heat. Add the chopped onion and garlic, and cook for 3 minutes or until the onions become translucent. Stir in the cinnamon stick and cook for an additional minute, stirring frequently. Add the passata, molasses, Dijon mustard, cooked soybeans, and vegetable stock to the saucepan. Bring the mixture to a boil.

5. Reduce the heat to low, cover the pan, and simmer gently for 1 hour, allowing the flavors to meld together. Stir the mixture once and add more vegetable stock if needed.

6. Stir in the apple cider vinegar and tamari soy sauce. Remove the cinnamon stick.

7. Serve the spicy soybeans spooned over the baked potatoes.

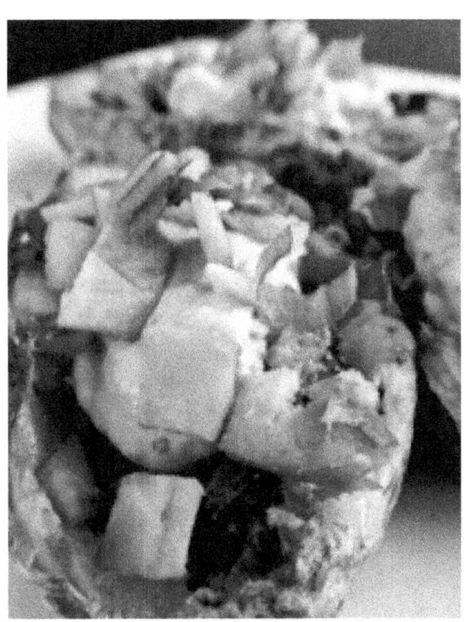

Potato Skins with Broccoli & Tofu

Prep Time	Cook Time	Servings
15 min	1hr. 30 min	4

INGREDIENTS:

- 1 tbsp sunflower oil
- 2 finely chopped onions
- 1 cup chopped mushrooms
- ¼ tsp ground nutmeg
- 10 oz tofu

Method:

11. Preheat the oven to 200°C/400°F/Gas 6. Place the potatoes on a baking sheet and bake for 1 hour or until they are cooked.

12. Place the broccoli in a steamer over high heat and steam for 6 minutes until tender but still vibrant green. Remove from the steamer and set aside.

149

- 1 tbsp Dijon mustard

- Freshly ground black

  pepper

- 1 ¾ cups broccoli, cut

into florets

- 1 handful parsley, finely

chopped

- 4 large scrubbed and

scored baking/Idaho

potatoes

For serving:

- Salad

Nutritional Value:

- Calories: 314

- Carbohydrates: 42.6 g

- Protein: 14.3 g

- Fat: 10.2 g

-

13. Heat the sunflower oil in a frying pan over low heat. Add the chopped onions and cook, stirring occasionally, for 3 minutes or until they become translucent. Add the mushrooms and cook for another 5 minutes, stirring often. Season with ground nutmeg and black pepper. Remove from heat.

14. Slice the baked potatoes in half lengthwise and scoop out the insides, leaving a thick shell of potato skin. Combine the scooped-out potato, steamed broccoli, tofu, parsley, and Dijon mustard in a mixing bowl. Mash the ingredients together until a smooth mixture is formed. Add the cooked mushrooms and onions, and stir to combine.

15. Spoon the mixture back into the potato skins.

16. Return the filled potato skins to the oven and bake for 15 minutes or until heated.

17. Serve the potato skins immediately with a side of salad.

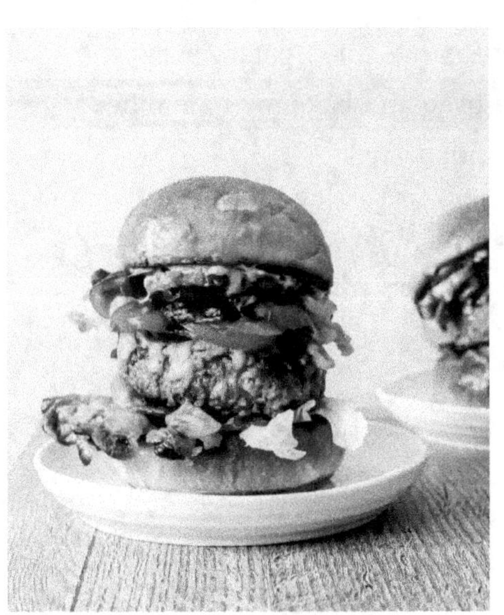

Bean Burgers

Prep Time	Cook Time	Servings
10 min	1 hr	2

INGREDIENTS:

- 2 garlic cloves, crushed

- 1 onion, finely chopped

- 2 tomatoes, finely chopped

- 1 tsp black pepper

Method:

1. Put the beans in a large bowl, cover them with cold water, and leave to soak overnight or for at least 12 hours.

2. Drain the beans and rinse thoroughly. Put them in a large saucepan, cover them with cold water, and boil over high heat. Boil for 10 minutes, then reduce the heat to low. Cover with a lid and let it simmer for 1 hour or until the beans are soft. Drain the

- ½ tsp chili powder
- 1 tbsp sunflower oil
- Freshly ground

black pepper

- ½ cup mixed dried

beans (such as butter

beans, soybeans,

or black-eyed beans)

For srving:

- Salad

Nutritional Value:

- Calories: 233
- Carbohydrates: 27.1 g
- Protein: 11.6 g
- Fat: 8.8 g

beans, mash them well to make a thick paste, and let them cool.

3. Transfer the mashed beans to a serving bowl and stir in the crushed garlic, finely chopped onion, tomatoes, black pepper, and chili powder. Divide the mixture into 8 equal portions and shape each into a ball using your hands. Flatten the balls to form burger patties.

4. Heat half the sunflower oil in a frying pan over medium heat until hot. Add half of the burger patties and fry them for 5 minutes on each side until browned. Keep the cooked burgers warm while you cook the remaining ones, adding the remaining oil as necessary.

5. Serve the bean burgers with a side of salad.

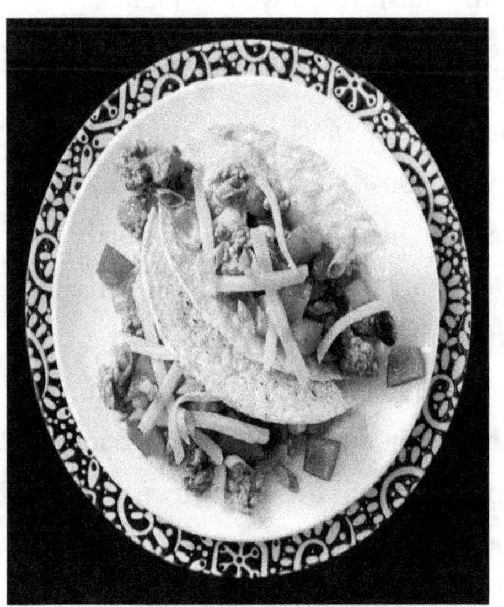

Bean Tacos

Prep Time   Cook Time   Servings

25 min   10 min   6

INGREDIENTS:

- 1 tbsp soy oil
- 1 onion, finely chopped
- 4 tomatoes, diced
- 2 tbsp soy yogurt
- ¾ cup soy mince/ground

"meat" TVP

- ½ tsp Chinese five spice
- ½ tsp chili powder
-

Method:

6. Put the soy mince/TVP in a small heatproof bowl and pour in ½ cup boiling water. Leave it to stand for 10-15 minutes until the water has been absorbed. Rinse and drain thoroughly.

7. Stir the five Chinese spices into the soy yogurt and set it aside.

8. Heat the soy oil in a frying pan over medium heat. Add the chopped onion and green pepper

- 1 deseeded & finely chopped green pepper

- 2 tbsp tomato purée /paste

- 3 ¼ cups drained & rinsed canned mixed beans

(e.g., kidney beans & black-eyed beans)

- 8 taco shells
- 8 large shredded lettuce leaves
- 2 avocados, peeled, pitted, & diced

Nutritional Value:

- Calories: 267
- Carbohydrates: 34.3 g
- Protein: 22.7 g
- Fat: 4.3 g
-

and fry, stirring occasionally, for about 3 minutes or until tender. Add the tomato purée/paste, mixed beans, soy mince/TVP, and the spicy yogurt mixture. Pour in ¼ cup water. Cook for 6 minutes or until the beans have softened.

9. Remove the pan from the heat. Spoon the bean mixture into the taco shells.

10.

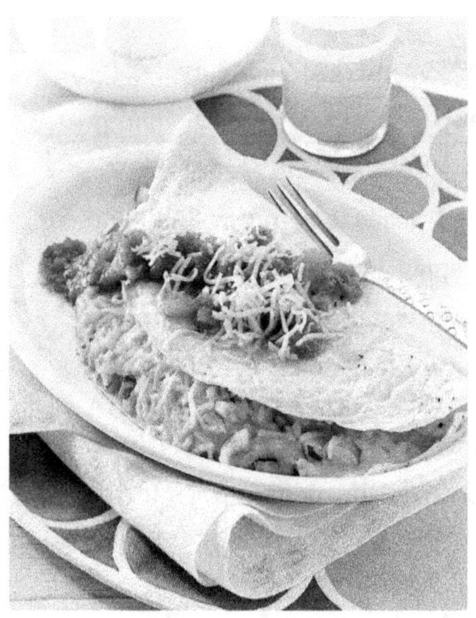

Spanish Omelet

Prep Time	Cook Time	Servings
15 min	30 min	6

INGREDIENTS:

- 2 garlic cloves,
- 6 eggs
- 2 tbsp olive oil
- 3 small sliced

potatoes

- ½ cup unsweetened

soy milk

Method:

1. Heat the olive oil in a large, ovenproof, non-stick frying pan over medium heat. Add the sliced potatoes and red pepper. Cover the pan with a lid and fry for about 10 minutes, or until the potatoes are cooked, stirring occasionally. Add the sliced onion and bacon, and cook for 10 minutes or until the bacon is cooked, stirring frequently. Stir in the chopped oregano and season with black pepper.

156

- ½ tsp chili powder
- 1red onion, halved &

thinly sliced

- 1 red pepper, deseeded

& cut into strips

- 2 rindless bacon slices,

cut into strips

- 1 finely chopped small

handful of oregano leaves

- Freshly ground black

pepper

For serving:

- Salad

Nutritional Value:

- Calories: 208
- Carbohydrates: 14.1 g
- Protein: 10.3 g
- Fat: 12.3 g

2. Preheat the grill/broiler to medium. In a jug, whisk together the eggs and soy milk. Pour the egg mixture over the cooked ingredients in the frying pan. Cover the pan again and cook over medium heat for about 5 minutes or until the bottom is golden and set.

3. Remove the pan from the heat and place it under the preheated grill/broiler for another 10 minutes or until the top is golden. Serve the Spanish omelet warm with a side of salad.

11.

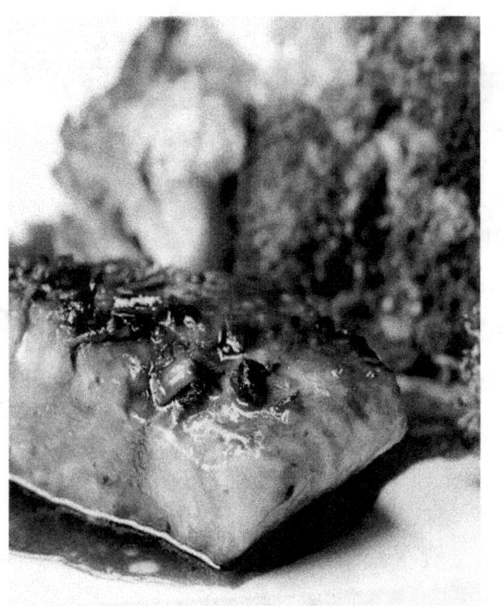

Salmon with Honey Soy Glaze

Prep Time	Cook Time	Servings
5 min	15-20 min	4

INGREDIENTS:

- 4 salmon fillets
- (approximately 150 g)
- 4 tbsp tamari soy sauce
- 2 tsp sesame oil
- 1 tbsp clear honey
- 2 tbsp mirin
- 4 tsp grated ginger

Method:

1. Preheat the oven to 425°F/Gas 7. Place the salmon fillets in a shallow baking dish.

2. Mix the honey, sesame oil, mirin, tamari soy sauce, and grated ginger until well combined. Pour the mixture evenly over the salmon fillets, ensuring they are well coated.

For serving:

- Steamed tender-stem broccoli, asparagus, or bok choy

3. Bake the salmon in the oven for 15-20 minutes, or until the salmon is cooked and flakes easily with a knife.

4. Serve warm salmon with steamed tender-stem broccoli, asparagus, or bok choy. Alternatively, you can enjoy it cold as part of a salad.

Nutritional Value:

- Calories: 369
- Carbohydrates: 5.5 g
- Protein: 29.8 g
- Fat: 25.4 g

4.

Kale, Chicken and Parmesan Bowl

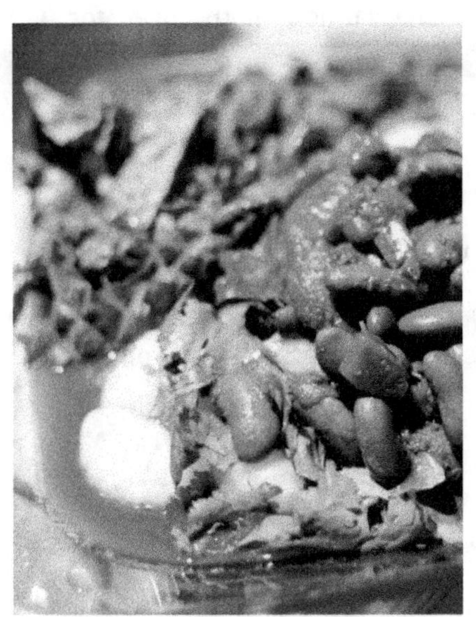

Prep Time	Cook Time	Servings
5 min	25 min	4

INGREDIENTS:

- 4 salmon fillets
- 2 tbsp olive oil
- 4 cups skinless

chicken breast

(cut into smaller fillets)

- 4 garlic cloves, thinly

sliced

- 1 cup roughly grated

Parmesan

-

Method:

1. Heat a large frying pan over medium heat. Add half of the olive oil and the chopped kale. Toss the kale for a few minutes until wilted. Remove the wilted kale from the pan and set it aside.

2. Heat the remaining olive oil in the same pan and add the chicken fillets. Stir until the chicken is cooked through and golden brown. Remove the cooked

160

- 3 ¼ cups stems removed

& chopped kale

- 2 tbsp rinsed pine nuts
- Juice of 1 lemon

Nutritional Value:

- Calories: 332

- Carbohydrates: 4.3 g

- Protein: 40.8 g

- Fat: 16.9 g

chicken from the pan and set it aside.

3. Add the garlic and pine nuts to the pan and stir for 1-2 minutes until the garlic is golden brown and fragrant. Return the wilted kale and cooked chicken to the pan.

4. Pour the lemon juice over the ingredients in the pan and sprinkle the grated Parmesan. Toss everything together to combine all the ingredients well.

5. Serve the kale, chicken, and Parmesan bowl immediately.

5.

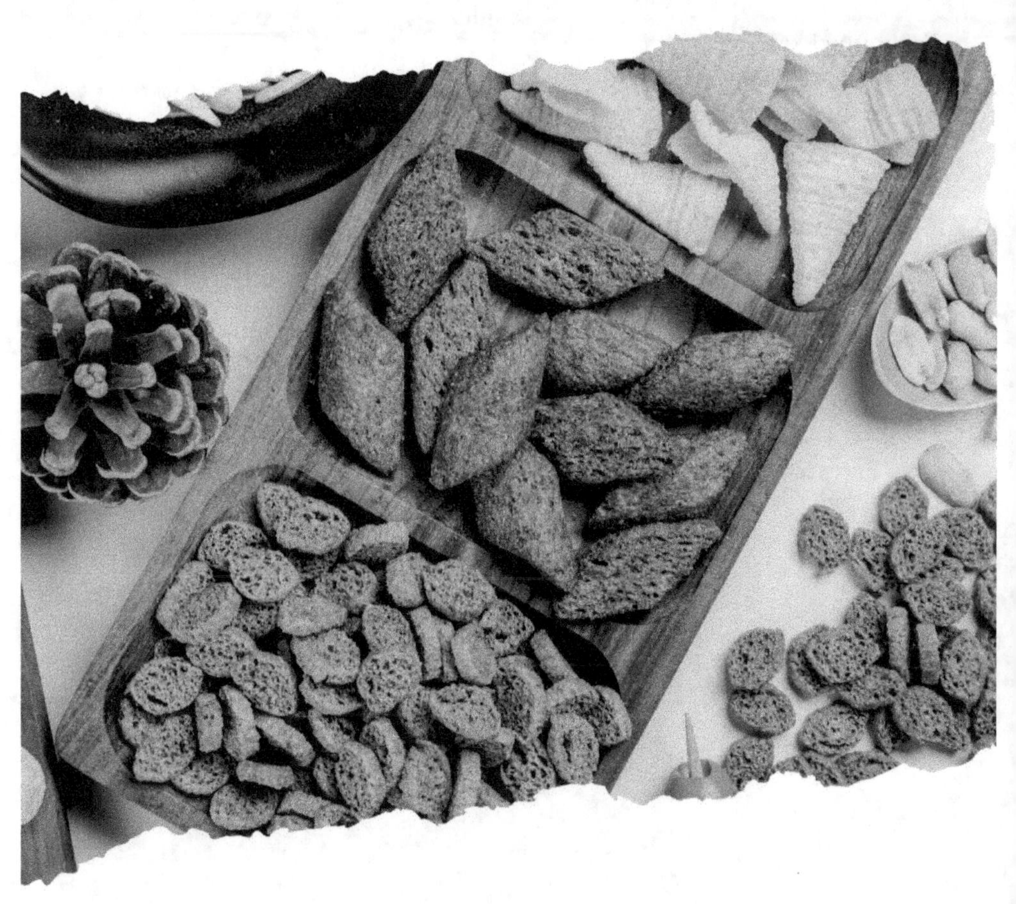

Snack Recipes

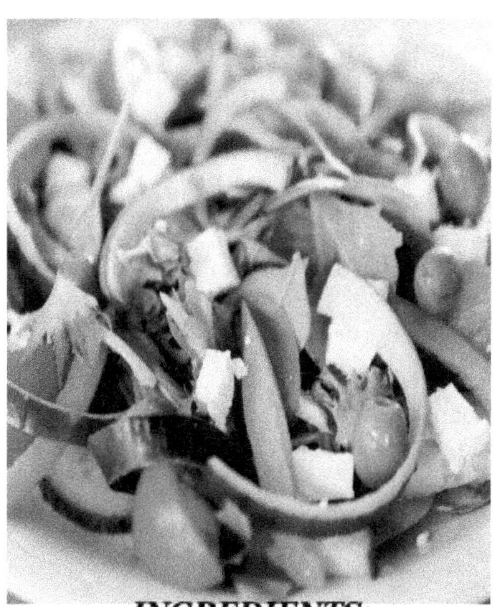

Apple & Nut Salad

Prep Time	Cook Time	Servings
10 min	None	4

INGREDIENTS:

- 4 red apples peeled, quartered, & cored
- Juice of ½ lemon
- ½ cucumber, cut into batons
- 6 celery sticks, chopped
- 1 bunch spring onions /scallions, sliced
- ½ cup unroasted, salt-free
- peanuts

Method:

1. Cut each apple quarter into 3 slices and dip them into the lemon juice to prevent discoloration.

2. Place the apple slices in a serving bowl. Add the cucumber batons, chopped celery sticks, sliced spring onions/scallions, and unroasted peanuts.

3. Mix all the ingredients in the bowl.

163

For serving:

4. Serve the Apple & Nut Salad with your choice of salad dressing.

- Salad dressing

Nutritional Value:

- Calories: 170
- Carbohydrates: 13.8 g
- Protein: 6.7 g
- Fat: 9.9 g
-

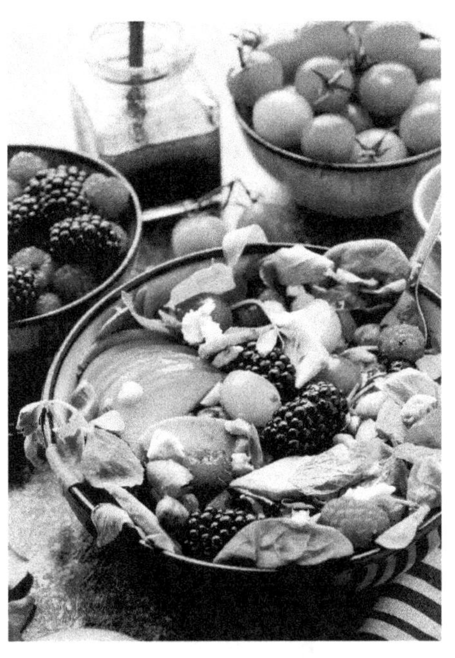

Fruit & Nut Salad

Prep Time	Cook Time	Servings
15 min	None	4

INGREDIENTS:

- 4 red apples peeled,
- 3 oranges
- ¼ cup walnuts,

chopped

- ¼ cup almonds,

flaked/sliced

- 2 apples, cored and

cut into wedges

Method:

1. Place the torn leaves of curly endive/chicory lettuce in a salad bowl.

2. In a separate large bowl, grate the zest of 1 orange. Peel the oranges and break the flesh into segments. Add the orange segments to the bowl with the grated zest. Also, add the flaked/sliced almonds, chopped walnuts, apple wedges, grapes, and lemon juice. Mix well to combine.

165

- ¾ cup seedless grapes
- 1 tbsp lemon juice
- 2 heads of curly

endive/chicory

lettuce (leaves torn

into pieces)

Nutritional Value:

- Calories: 171

- Carbohydrates: 22.8 g

- Protein: 4 g

- Fat: 7.1 g

-

3. Pour the fruit and nut mixture into the salad bowl's endive/chicory leaves.

4. Chill the salad in the refrigerator for 10 minutes.

5. Serve the Endive, Fruit & Nut Salad chilled.

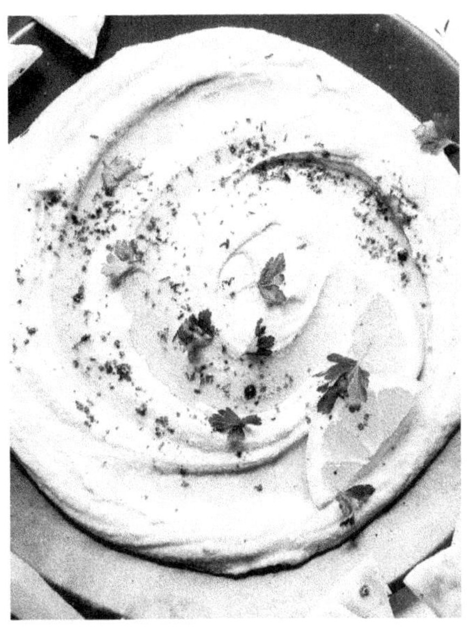

Hummus

Prep Time	Cook Time	Servings
15 min	1-1 ½ hr.	6

INGREDIENTS:

- 1 cup dried chickpeas
- 1 cup sesame seeds
- 2 tbsp tahini
- 2 tbsp soy oil
- 5 garlic cloves
- Juice of 3 lemons
- Pinch of paprika
- (optional)

Method:

1. Place the dried chickpeas in a bowl, cover them with cold water, and let them soak overnight or for at least 12 hours.

2. Drain and rinse the soaked chickpeas thoroughly. Transfer them to a saucepan, cover them with fresh cold water, and boil over high heat. Boil for 10 minutes, then reduce the heat to low. Cover the saucepan with a lid and let it simmer for 1-1 ½ hours

For serving:

- Rice cakes

Nutritional Value:

- Calories: 298
- Carbohydrates: 24g
- Protein: 11.3 g
- Fat: 17.5 g

until the chickpeas are tender. Drain and let them cool.

3. Combine the sesame seeds, tahini, soy oil, garlic cloves, and half of the lemon juice in a blender or food processor. Blend until smooth.

4. Add the cooked and cooled chickpeas and lemon juice to the blender or food processor. Continue blending until the mixture becomes smooth and creamy.

5. For a touch of spiciness, add a pinch of paprika if desired.

6. Serve the hummus with rice cakes or your preferred accompaniments.

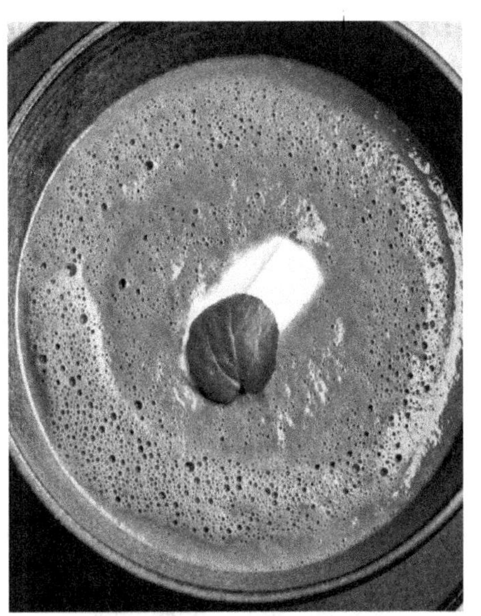

INGREDIENTS:

- ½ cup soy margarine
- 4 cups vegetable stock
- 6 potatoes, diced
- 1 onion, finely chopped
- Pinch of ground nutmeg
- 6 bunches trimmed

watercress (plus extra

for garnish)

- Freshly ground black

pepper

Watercress Soup

Prep Time   Cook Time   Servings

5 min   30 min   8

Method:

1. In a frying pan, melt the soy margarine over low heat. Add the chopped onion and sauté gently for about 5 minutes, until the onion turns transparent.

2. Add the diced potatoes, vegetable stock, and ground nutmeg to the pan. Cover with a lid and let it simmer for 15 minutes or until the potatoes are cooked and tender.

3. Add the watercress to the pan and continue simmering for another

169

Nutritional Value:

- Calories: 24 g

- Carbohydrates: 27.9 g

- Protein: 4.1 g

- Fat: 12.7 g

10 minutes, allowing the flavors to blend.

4. Let the soup cool for about 10 minutes. Then, transfer it to a blender or food processor and blend until smooth and creamy.

5. Season the soup with freshly ground black pepper according to taste.

6. Serve the soup in bowls, garnished with a sprig of watercress.

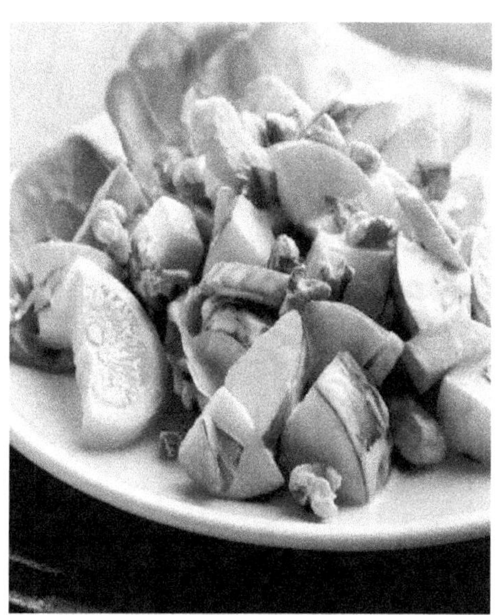

Apple, Celery and Beetroot Salad

Prep Time	Cook Time	Servings
5 min	30 min	8

INGREDIENTS:

- 2 celery stalks, diced
- 2 tbsp walnuts, chopped
- 2 large beetroot/beets, peeled & sliced

Method:

1. Place the beetroot/beets in a steamer and steam over medium heat for about 20 minutes or until tender. Transfer the steamed beetroot to a serving bowl and let it cool.

2. Mix the apple wedges, diced celery, and chopped walnuts in the same serving bowl.

3. Combine the Dijon mustard, clear honey, and mayonnaise in a small

Nutritional Value:

- Calories: 259
- Carbohydrates:

14.5 g

- Protein: 2.5 g
- Fat: 21.3 g

French dressing:

- 1 tbsp Dijon mustard
- 4 tbsp extra virgin

olive oil

- 2 tbsp white wine vinegar
- 1 tbsp clear honey
- 2 apples, cored & cut into wedges
- 1 tbsp mayonnaise
- Freshly ground black pepper

mixing bowl to make the dressing. In a separate jug, mix the olive oil and white wine vinegar. Slowly add the oil and vinegar mixture to the mustard mixture while whisking continuously with a hand whisk until the dressing is smooth.

4. Pour the dressing over the salad in the serving bowl. Season with freshly ground black pepper according to taste.

5. Serve the salad immediately.

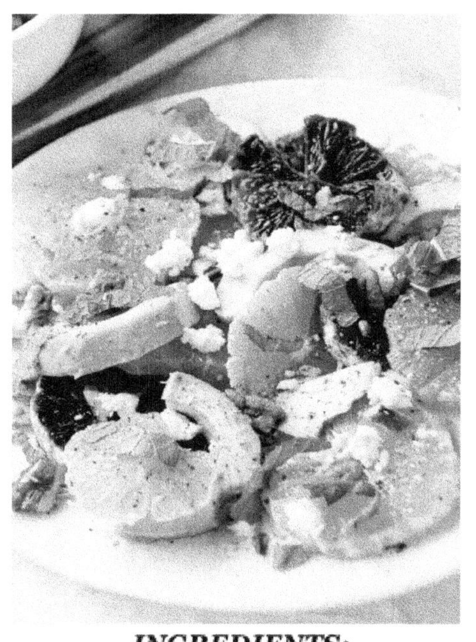

Orange & Avocado Salad

  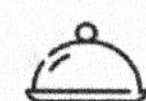

Prep Time	Cook Time	Servings
10 min	None	4

INGREDIENTS:

- 4 tomatoes, sliced
- 12 lettuce leaves
- 2 avocados, peeled,
- pitted, & chopped
- 4 oranges, peeled
- & separated into

segments

- 2 spring onions/scallions,
- finely chopped

Method:

6. Combine the chopped avocados, sliced tomatoes, orange segments, spring onions/scallions, and lettuce leaves in a serving bowl.

7. Whisk together the lemon juice, orange juice, flaxseed oil, and finely chopped ginger to make the dressing in a separate jug.

8. Pour the dressing over the salad in the serving bowl.

173

Nutritional Value:

- Calories: 259

- Calories: 331

- Carbohydrates: 19.3 g

- Protein: 6.5 g

- Fat: 25 g

French dressing:

- 2 tbsp orange juice

- 2 tbsp lemon juice

- 2 tsp flaxseed oil

- ½ in piece of peeled

& finely chopped root ginger

9. Mix all the ingredients until well combined.

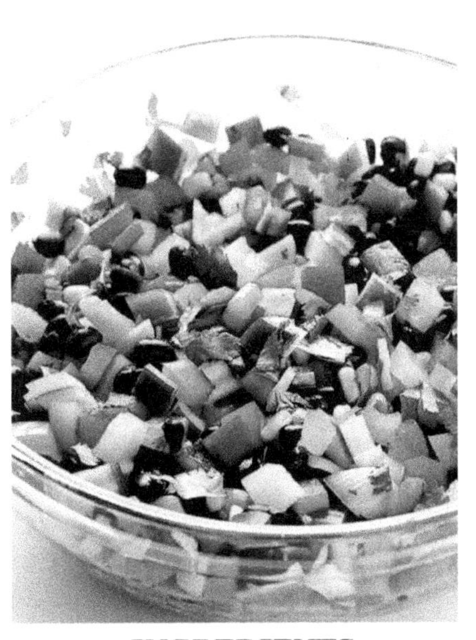

Rainbow Salsa

Prep Time	Cook Time	Servings
15 min	1 hr	4

INGREDIENTS:

- 1 large ripe mango, peeled & diced

- 1 cucumber, diced

- 1 small red onion, finely diced

- 1 red pepper, deseeded & finely diced

Method:

1. In a large bowl, combine all the ingredients.

2. Stir well to thoroughly combine everything.

3. Refrigerate the salsa for at least 1 hour to allow the flavors to develop.

4. Enjoy the rainbow salsa with your favorite chips, tacos, or as a refreshing side dish.

- 1 avocado, pitted and
- diced
- 1 large tomato, finely diced
- 2 garlic cloves, finely chopped
- 1 tbsp scant flat-leaf parsley or coriander, chopped
- ½ tsp sea salt
- 2 tbsp extra virgin olive oil
- Juice of 2 limes

Nutritional Value:

- Calories: 237
- Carbohydrates: 18.2 g
- Protein: 3.4 g
- Fat: 16.7 g

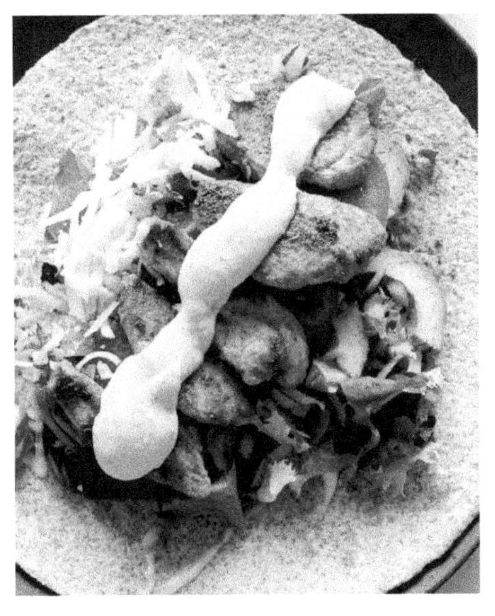

Sardine and Avocado Wrap

Prep Time	Cook Time	Servings
10 min	1 hr	8

INGREDIENTS:

- 16 black pitted and halved olives
- Juice of 1-2 lemons
- 20 strands chives, chopped
- 2 cups can whole sardines in olive oil, drained

Method:

1. In a bowl, gently break the sardines into chunks.

2. Add half of the avocado, black olives, lemon juice, and chopped chives to the bowl.

3. Toss the ingredients together until well combined.

4. Refrigerate the mixture for 1 hour to allow the flavors to meld.

- 2 small pitted & sliced or diced avocados

- 1 large head of green chicory (leaves separated)

Nutritional Value:

- Calories: 248

- Carbohydrates: 1.3 g

- Protein: 15 g

- Fat: 20.2 g

5. Fill each leaf of green chicory with the sardine and avocado mixture, dividing it evenly.

6. Top the wraps with the remaining avocado slices.

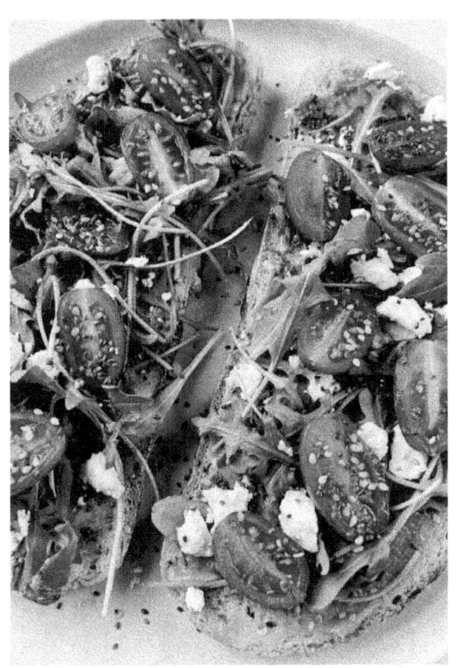

INGREDIENTS:

- 2 garlic cloves

- 2 tomatoes

- 4 bread slices (ideally gluten-free)

- 1-2 tbsp extra virgin olive oil

- Sea salt and freshly ground black pepper

Tomato and Garlic Toast

Prep Time   Cook Time   Servings

10 min   10 min   4

Method:

1. Toast the bread on both sides until lightly brown and crunchy.

2. Peel the garlic cloves five minutes before using them to allow the antibacterial compound allicin to form, maximizing its benefits.

Option 1 (milder garlic flavor):

1. Finely grate the tomatoes into a bowl.

179

Nutritional Value:

- Calories: 166
- Carbohydrates: 21.3 g
- Protein: 2.9 g
- Fat: 7.5 g

2. Cut the garlic cloves in half and rub them over the toasted bread.

3. Spoon the grated tomato over the garlicky toast.

4. Drizzle with a splash of olive oil and season with salt and pepper.

Option 2 (stronger garlic flavor):

1. Finely grate the tomatoes into a bowl.

2. Crush or grate the garlic cloves and add them to the tomatoes.

3. Add the olive oil, season with salt and pepper, and mix well.

4. Spoon the tomato mixture over the toasted bread.

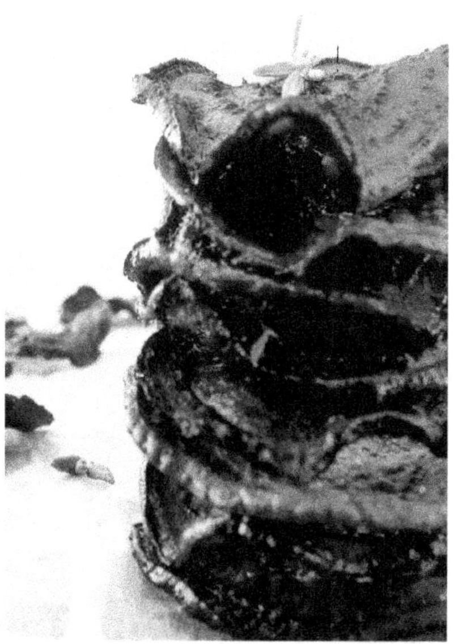

Beetroot Crisps

Prep Time	Cook Time	Servings
10 min	15-20 min	4

INGREDIENTS:

- 12 oz beetroot, peeled

- 3 tbsp extra virgin olive oil

- 1 tsp sea salt

- 2-3 tbsp rosemary, roughly chopped

- Hummus, to serve (optional)

Method:

1. Preheat the oven to 400°F/Gas 6. Use a food processor to slice the beetroot into consistent slices, ensuring even baking and crispness.

2. Combine the olive oil, sea salt, and rosemary in a large bowl.

3. Add the beetroot slices to the bowl and use a brush to coat them evenly with the oil mixture. Gently turn the slices to ensure they are well coated.

181

Nutritional Value:

- Calories: 131

- Carbohydrates: 5.1 g

- Protein: 1.1 g

- Fat: 11.7 g

4. Arrange the beetroot slices in a single layer on two baking trays. The slices can touch, but make sure they don't overlap.

5. Bake the trays in the center of the oven for 15-20 minutes, depending on the thickness of the slices. Keep a close eye on them after 10 minutes, as they can quickly burn.

6. Remove the trays from the oven and let the beetroot chips cool on a wire rack until they become crispy.

7. Serve the beetroot chips as a healthy snack, or enjoy them with hummus if desired.

8. Note: The beetroot chips can be stored in an airtight container for a few days.

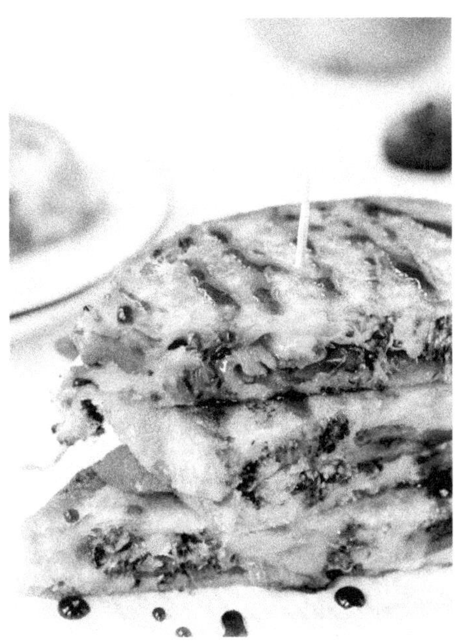

Broccoli Bread

Prep Time	Cook Time	Servings
20 min	1 hr	10

Method:

INGREDIENTS:

- 3 ¼ cups steamed broccoli, blended
- ¾ cup ground flaxseeds
- 3 tbsp coconut oil
- ¼ tsp freshly ground black pepper
- ¼ tsp sea salt
- 1 tsp baking powder
- 2 tbsp chia seeds

1. Preheat the oven to 400°F/Gas 6. Line a loaf tin measuring 8 x 4 inches with parchment paper.

2. Combine the blended broccoli, ground flaxseeds, chia seeds, coconut flour, chickpea flour, coconut oil, black pepper, sea salt, baking powder, almond milk, chopped basil, and pumpkin seeds in a large bowl. Mix well until they form a dough-like consistency.

183

- 1 ½ tbsp coconut flour
- 1 ½ tbsp chickpea

(gram) flour

- ½ cup almond milk
- 1 ½ tbsp pumpkin

seeds

- ½ tbsp basil, chopped

Nutritional Value:

- Calories: 147
- Carbohydrates: 6 g
- Protein: 3.8 g
- Fat: 11.9 g

3. Place the dough in the loaf tin and bake for 1 hour or until cooked through and an inserted skewer comes out clean.

4. Leave the bread to cool in the tin before serving.

5. Enjoy the bread warm, or let it cool completely and toast it.

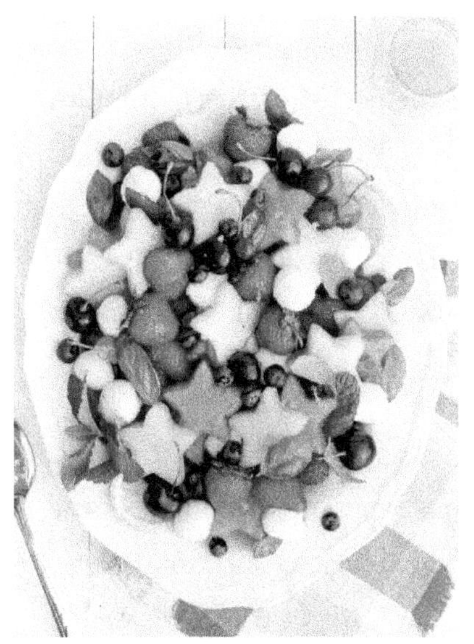

Ginger Fruit Salad

Prep Time	Cook Time	Servings
20 min	10 min	4

INGREDIENTS:

- 3 tbsp syrup
- 2 lb honeydew melon
- 1 tbsp soft light brown sugar

- 2 oranges, peeled & pith removed

- 3 apples, peeled, cored, & chopped

- Juice of 2 oranges
- 2 pieces jarred preserved stem ginger, finely chopped

Method:

1. Combine the orange juice, chopped stem ginger, ginger syrup, and brown sugar in a saucepan. Heat gently over low heat for 3-4 minutes until the sugar has dissolved. Increase the heat to medium-high, bring the mixture to a boil, and cook for 5 minutes or until it becomes syrupy. Remove from heat and let it cool for 10 minutes.

2. Slice the peeled oranges into thick rings and then cut the rings into quarters, removing any seeds. Cut the honeydew melon in half, remove the seeds, and scoop out the flesh.

3. Place all the fruit (oranges, melons, and chopped apples) in a serving bowl. Pour the ginger syrup over the fruit and stir well to coat. Cover the bowl with cling film/plastic wrap and refrigerate for 1-2 hours to allow the flavors to meld.

4. Before serving, sprinkle fresh mint leaves over the top of the fruit salad.

5. Feel free to add other fruits of your choice, such as grapes or berries, to enhance the variety of flavors.

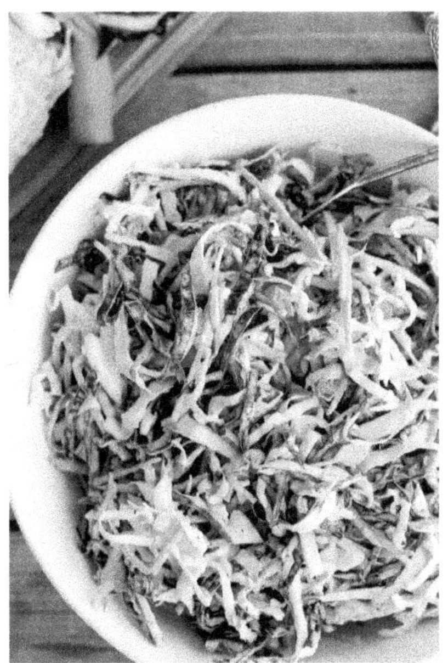

Coleslaw

Prep Time	Cook Time	Servings
10 min	None	4

INGREDIENTS:

- 3 tbsp syrup
- 5 carrots, coarsely grated
- 1 large apple, coarsely grated
- ½ cup scant raisins
- 4 tbsp soy yogurt

Method:

1. Combine the shredded cabbage, grated carrots, apple, and raisins in a serving bowl.

2. In a small jug, whisk together the soy yogurt and soy mayonnaise. Season with freshly ground black pepper.

3. Pour the dressing over the salad and mix well to ensure all the ingredients are coated.

4. Serve and enjoy!

187

- 4 tbsp soy mayonnaise
- 1 white cabbage cored

& finely shredded

- Freshly ground black

pepper

Nutritional Value:

- Calories: 210
- Carbohydrates: 26.9 g
- Protein: 5.2g
- Fat: 9 g

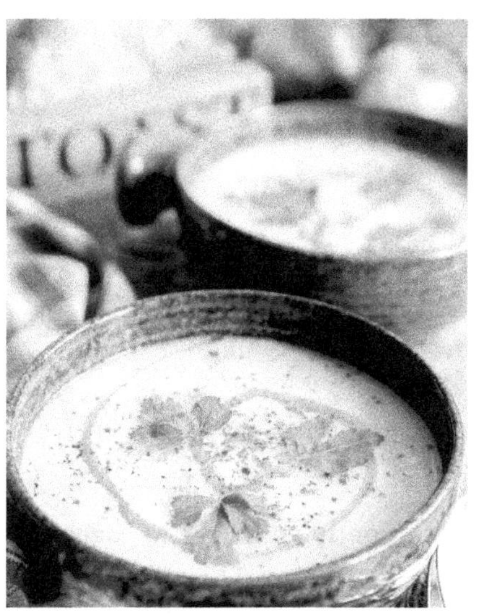

Parsnip & Apple Soup

Prep Time	Cook Time	Servings
10 min	30 min	4

INGREDIENTS:

- 3 tbsp syrup
- 1 tsp olive oil
- 1 onion, diced
- 6 large parsnips,

peeled & roughly

chopped

- 1 cooking apple peeled,

cored, & roughly

chopped

Method:

1. Heat the olive oil in a saucepan over medium-low heat. Add the diced onion and sauté for about 3 minutes until translucent.

2. Add the chopped parsnips and apple to the saucepan, then pour in the vegetable stock. Heat the mixture over medium heat until it reaches boiling point, then lower the heat to a gentle level and cover it with a lid, let it simmer for 30

- ¾ cup vegetable stock

- ⅔ scant cup skimmed milk

- Freshly ground black

pepper

Nutritional Value:

- Calories: 130

- Carbohydrates: 14 g

- Protein: 5.4 g

- Fat: 3.5 g

minutes or until the parsnips are very soft.

3. Allow the soup to cool for 10 minutes, then transfer it to a blender or food processor. Blend until smooth.

4. Return the soup to the saucepan and stir in the skimmed milk. Reheat gently over low heat. Season with freshly ground black pepper.

5. Serve the soup hot, and enjoy!

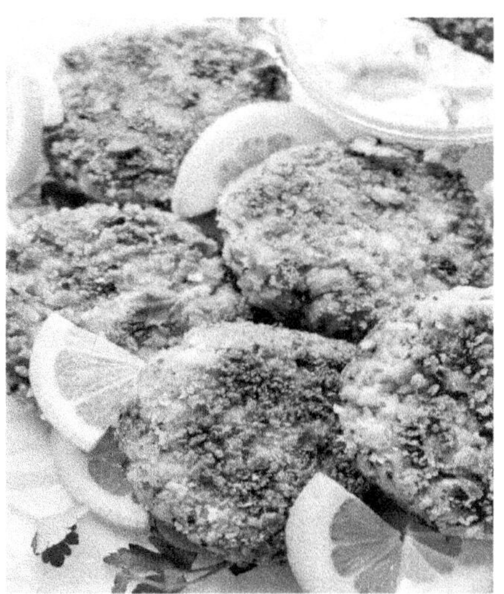

Black Olive and tuna Cake

Prep Time	Cook Time	Servings
10 min	40 min	10

INGREDIENTS:

- 3 tbsp syrup
- 3 eggs
- 1/3 cup olive oil
- 1 cup buckwheat flour
- 1 tsp baking powder
- 1 cup black pitted olives, rinsed
- 1 cup cheddar, grated
- 2 drained cans tuna
- 1/3 cup unsweetened milk of your choice

Method:

1. Preheat the oven to 400°F/Gas 6.

2. In a large bowl, combine the buckwheat flour and baking powder. Add the eggs and use a hand-held electric whisk to combine the ingredients.

3. Pour in the milk and olive oil, and continue whisking until the batter is well combined.

4. Add the black olives, grated cheddar, and drained tuna to the batter. Mix well using a spatula

191

Nutritional Value:

- Calories: 257

- Carbohydrates: 10.7 g

- Protein: 12 g

- Fat: 18.4 g

until all the ingredients are evenly distributed.

5. Pour the mixture into an 8 x 4 inches baking tin.

6. Bake in the oven for 40 minutes or until the cake is slightly golden and heated through.

7. Remove from the oven and allow the cake to cool slightly before slicing.

8. Serve the Black Olive and Tuna Cake warm, or enjoy it cold.

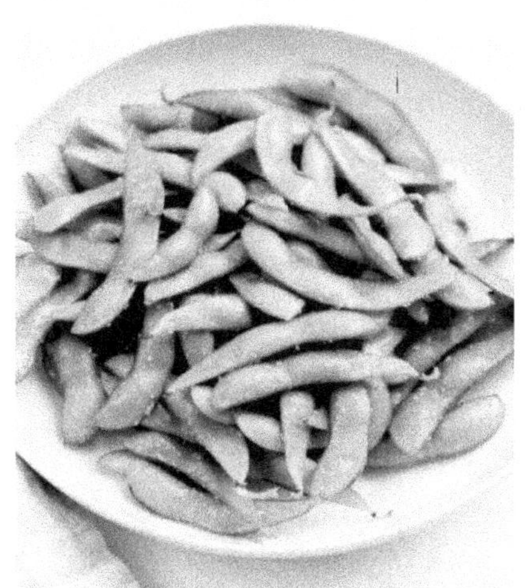

Edamame Beans

Prep Time	Cook Time	Servings
5 min	3-10 min	8

INGREDIENTS:

- 1 tsp extra virgin olive oil
- 2 lb frozen edamame with pods, or 1 lb without pods
- 1 garlic clove, crushed
- 2 tbsp grated Parmesan
- Sea salt flakes

Method:

1. Cook the edamame beans according to the package instructions.

2. Once cooked, drain the edamame beans and transfer them to a serving bowl.

3. Drizzle the extra virgin olive oil over the edamame beans.

4. Add the crushed garlic and toss to coat the beans evenly.

5. Sprinkle the grated Parmesan over the beans.

Nutritional Value:

- Calories: 172

- Carbohydrates: 11.3 g

- Protein: 13.2 g

- Fat: 8.1 g

6. Finish by sprinkling sea salt flakes over the top.

7. Enjoy the edamame beans as a snack or serve them as a side dish.

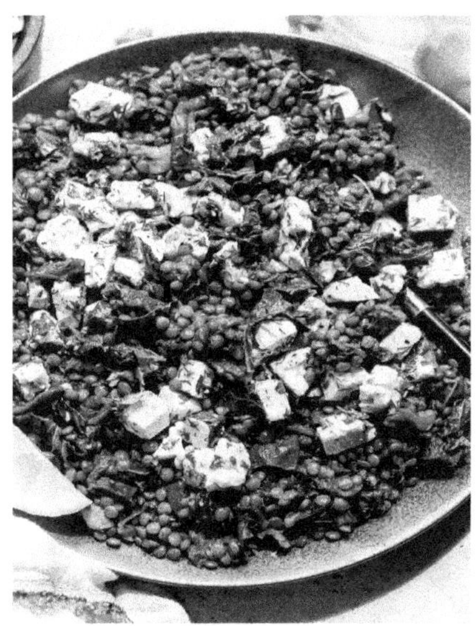

Puy Lentils, Ham & Feta Salad

Prep Time	Cook Time	Servings
1 5 min	15 min (rest 1-2 hr)	8

INGREDIENTS:

- 2 ¼ cups Puy lentils
- ½ cup sun-dried tomatoes
- 12 cherry tomatoes,

halved

- 1 red onion, thinly sliced
- 1 small cucumber, diced
- 1 cup feta cheese, diced

1 cup cooked ham hock,

shredded

- 1 yellow pepper, deseeded

& diced

Method:

1. Cook the Puy lentils according to the instructions on the packet. Once cooked, drain, cool, and set aside.

2. In a separate bowl, prepare the dressing by combining the lemon juice, lemon zest, olive oil, salt, and pepper. Set the dressing aside.

3. In a large serving bowl, add the cooked lentils, shredded ham hock, diced feta cheese, diced cucumber, diced yellow pepper,

195

- ½ cup black olives, pitted

and halved

- 1 tbsp flat-leaf parsley,

finely chopped

- Sea salt and freshly

ground black pepper

For the dressing:

- 3 tbsp olive oil
- Juice and zest of

2 lemons

- Sea salt and freshly

ground black pepper

Nutritional Value:

- Calories: 347
- Carbohydrates: 14.4 g
- Protein: 16.9 g
- Fat: 24.5 g

cherry tomatoes, red onion slices, halved black olives, sun-dried tomatoes, and chopped parsley.

4. Pour the dressing over the salad ingredients and carefully toss to combine all the flavors.

5. Serve the salad immediately or refrigerate it for 1-2 hours to allow the flavors to develop further.

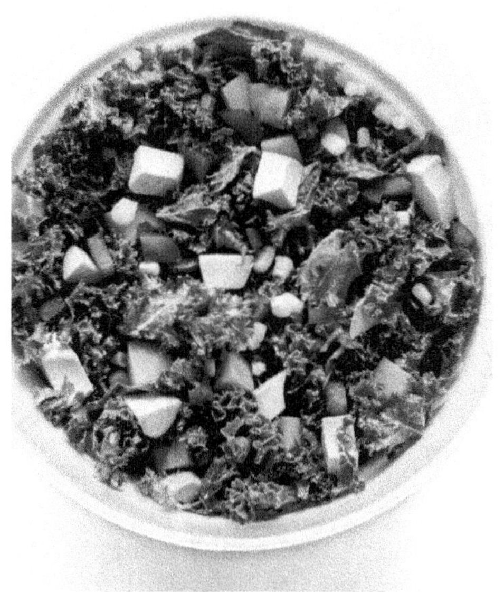

Magical Kale Salad

Prep Time	Cook Time	Servings
30 min	7 min(rest 1-2 hr)	4

INGREDIENTS:

- 2 cups kale, stalks removed
- 1 apple, cored & thinly sliced
- 1 tbsp olive oil
- 2 cups halloumi, sliced
- Juice of 1 lemon
- 1 ¾ oz flaked almonds
- ½ cup sunflower seeds
- ½ cup dried cranberries or sultanas
- Sea salt flakes (optional)

Method:

1. Blend all the dressing ingredients in a food processor until smooth to prepare the dressing.

2. Place the kale and apple in a large salad bowl. Pour the dressing over the salad and mix well, using your hands to massage and wilt the kale slightly. Refrigerate for 1-2 hours to allow the flavors to develop.

3. In a pan, heat the olive oil over medium heat. Add the halloumi slices and cook for about 3

For the dressing:

- 1 tbsp olive oil

- 1 tbsp sesame oil

- Juice of 1 lemon

- 2 tsp sumac

- 1 apple, cored & roughly

chopped

- 1 tbsp clear honey

- 3 tbsp tamari soy sauce

- 2 tsp ground cinnamon

- 1 2-in piece of fresh root

ginger, peeled and chopped

Nutritional Value:

- Calories: 308

- Carbohydrates: 21.4 g

- Protein: 7.5 g

- Fat: 22 g

minutes on each side until golden brown. Add the lemon juice to the pan and let it sizzle for 30 seconds. Turn the halloumi slices once more and set aside.

4. Arrange the halloumi slices on top of the dressed salad. Sprinkle with flaked almonds, sunflower seeds, dried cranberries or sultanas, and, if desired, some sea salt flakes.

5. Note: This salad can be a main course or a side dish.

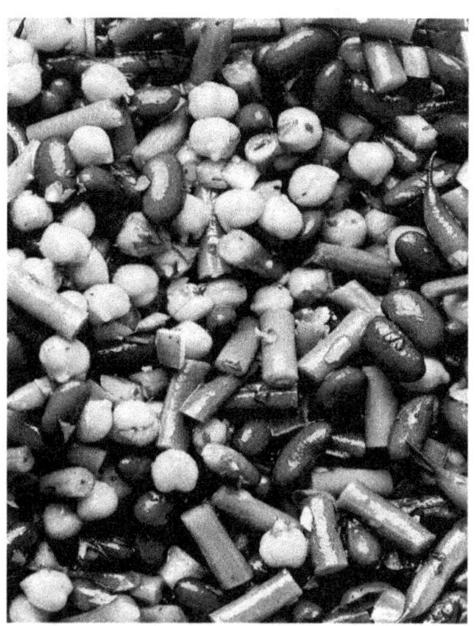

INGREDIENTS:

- 4 cups red kidney beans,

cooked

- 4 cups chickpeas, cooked

- 3 ¾ cups green beans,

cooked, cut into thirds

- 1 red onion, finely diced

- 1 tbsp flat-leaf parsley,

finely chopped

Three Bean Salad

Prep Time   Cook Time   Servings

15 min   5 min(rest 1 hr)   4

Method:

1. In a small bowl, combine all the dressing ingredients and stir well.

2. In a large bowl, combine the dressing, red kidney beans, chickpeas, green beans, diced red onion, and chopped parsley. Mix well to ensure all the ingredients are coated with the dressing.

3. Refrigerate the salad for 1 hour to allow the flavors to meld together.

4. Serve chilled and enjoy as a side dish or light meal.

For the dressing:

- 4 tbsp extra virgin olive oil

- 3 ¾ tbsp raw apple cider vinegar

- 1 tbsp wholegrain Dijon mustard

- Sea salt & freshly ground black pepper

Nutritional Value:

- Calories: 380

- Carbohydrates: 31.9 g

- Protein: 20.4 g

- Fat: 18.7 g

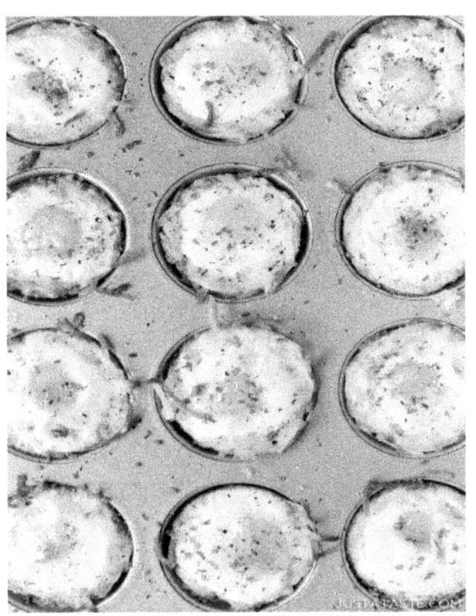

INGREDIENTS:

- 1 tsp butter

- 2 large eggs

- 1 ¼ oz smoked deli

ham or deli turkey,

diced

- ¼ cup cheddar cheese,

shredded

- Salt and freshly ground

black pepper

Easy Egg Cups

Prep Time   Cook Time   Servings

5 min   2 min   2

Method:

1. If not utilizing a microwave, preheat the oven to 400°F.

2. Grease one mug or ramekin per serving with butter.

3. Beat the eggs with a fork in the mug. Season with salt and pepper.

4. Add the diced ham and shredded cheese and mix thoroughly.

5. Microwave on high for 90 seconds to 2 minutes, or bake in the oven for 15 minutes until the cheese has melted and the eggs are firm.

Nutritional Value:

- Calories: 300
- Carbohydrates: 0.3 g
- Protein: 19.1 g
- Fat: 24.3 g

6. Allow the egg cup to cool slightly before serving.

8.

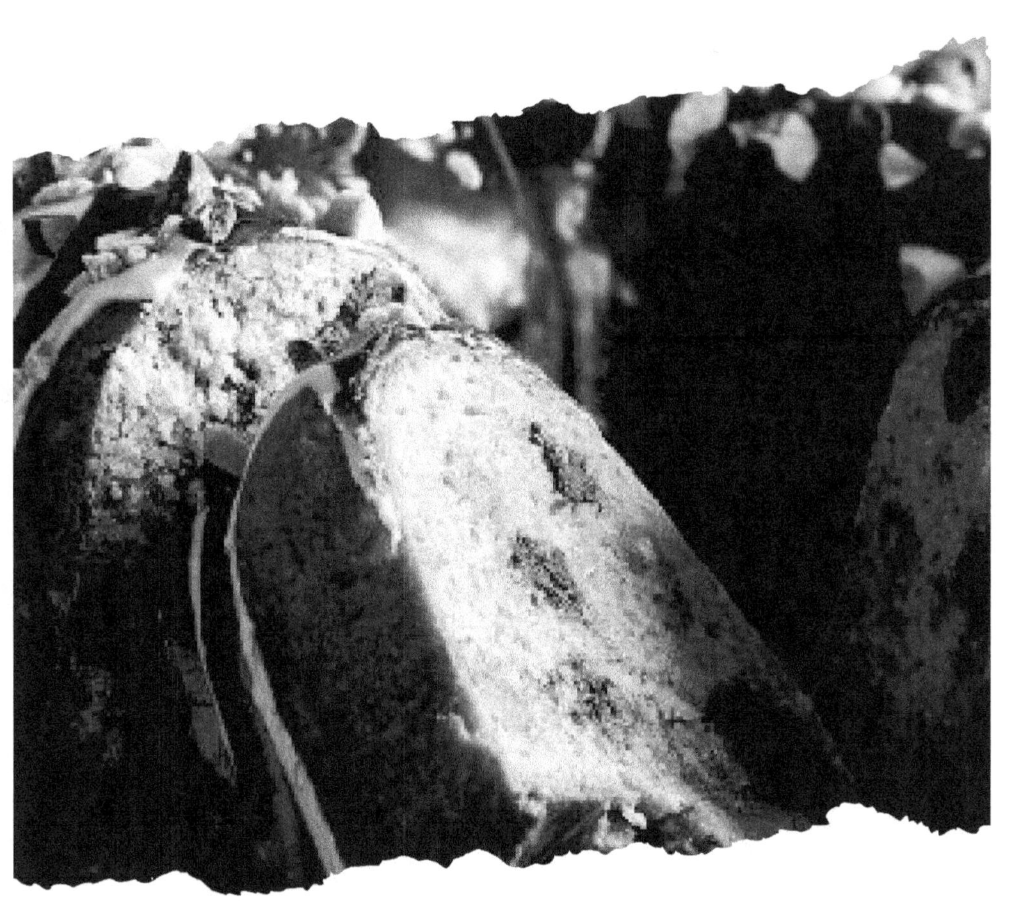

Dessert Recipes

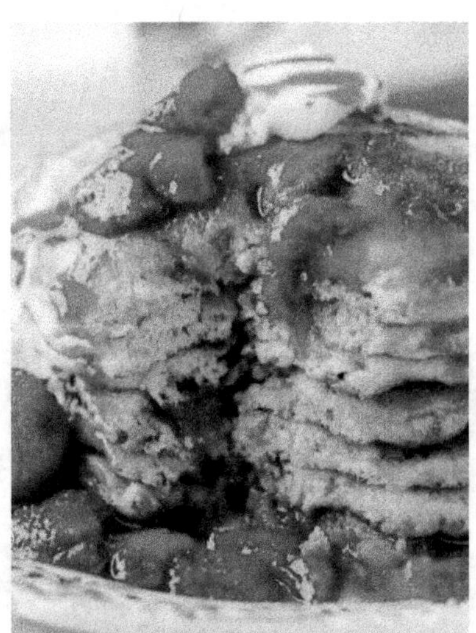

Strawberry Soufflé Pancakes

Prep Time	Cook Time	Servings
10 min	15 min	4

INGREDIENTS:

- Zest of 1 lemon
- 1 cup soy milk
- 2 separated eggs
- 1 tbsp caster/superfine sugar
- 1 tsp vanilla extract
- 3 tbsp clear honey
- 1 tbsp balsamic vinegar
- ¾ oz butter
- 4 cups strawberries, hulled & halved
- 1 ¼ scant cup self-rising flour

Method:

1. Whisk together the soy milk, egg yolks, lemon zest, flour, sugar, and vanilla extract in a large mixing bowl until smooth. Whisk the egg whites in a separate clean bowl until stiff peaks form. Gently fold the egg whites into the batter using a large metal spoon.

2. Combine the strawberries, honey, and balsamic vinegar in a bowl, mixing gently to coat the fruit.

3. Heat a little butter in a frying pan over medium heat until it melts.

For the dusting:

- Icing

- Confectioners' sugar

Nutritional Value:

- Calories: 233

- Carbohydrates: 28.4 g

- Protein: 7.6 g

- Fat: 8.7 g

Pour 2 tablespoons of the batter into the pan and tilt it to cover the bottom. Cook for 2 minutes until the underside is golden; flip the pancake with a spatula and cook for another 2 minutes until golden and puffed. Remove from the pan and keep warm. Repeat with the remaining batter.

4. Dust the pancakes with icing/confectioners' sugar and serve warm with the strawberries.

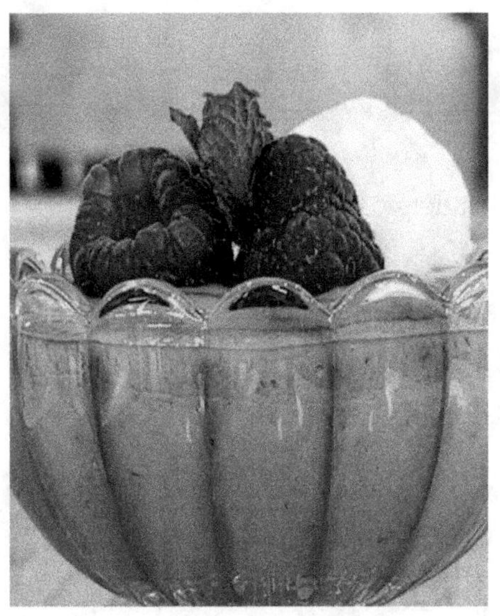

Raspberry & Tofu Brûlée

Prep Time | Cook Time | Servings

5 min | 3 min | 4

INGREDIENTS:

- 1 ⅔ scant cups

raspberries

- 9 oz silken tofu

- 2 tbsp clear honey

- 3 tbsp golden caster

/superfine sugar

Method:

1. Preheat the grill/broiler to high and grease 4 medium-sized ramekin dishes with sunflower oil.

2. Combine the raspberries, silken tofu, and honey in a blender or food processor. Blend until smooth.

3. Spoon the mixture into the greased ramekins and evenly sprinkle the sugar.

4. Place the ramekins under the grill/broiler for 2-3 minutes or

For greasing:

- Sunflower oil

Nutritional Value:

- Calories: 132

- Carbohydrates: 20.1 g

- Protein: 5.5 g

- Fat: 3 g

until a golden crust forms. Alternatively, you can use a blow torch to caramelize the sugar until it forms a hard, golden layer.

5. Serve the Raspberry & Tofu Brûlée immediately.

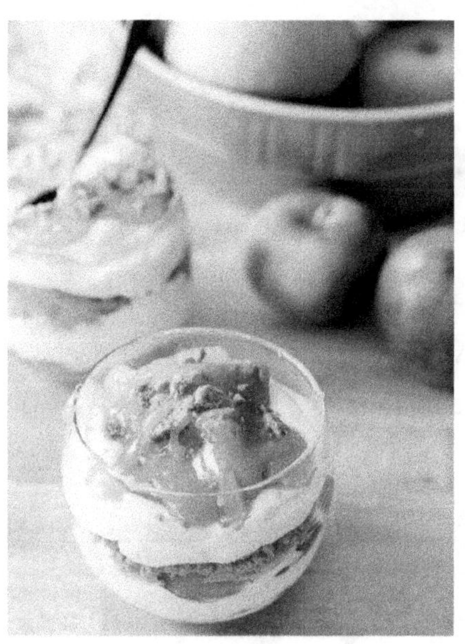

Apple & Tofu Cheesecake

Prep Time	Cook Time	Servings
20 min	40 min	10

INGREDIENTS:

- Seed Pastry

- ⅓ scant cup chopped

dried figs

- ¼ scant cup sunflower

seeds

- ¼ cup pumpkin seeds

- ½ tsp mixed/apple pie

spice

Method:

1. Preheat the oven to 350°F/Gas 4. Grease a 9-inch loose-bottom baking pan with soy margarine. The pan should be at least 3 ¼ inch deep.

2. Place the dried figs and 1 tablespoon of boiling water in a bowl. Let it stand for 10 minutes or until soft. Transfer to a blender or food processor and blend until smooth.

- ¼ cup toasted sesame seeds

- ¼ scant cup ground hazelnuts

Filling:

- 1 lb apples, peeled, cored, & chopped

- 2 tbsp lemon juice
- 1 tsp vanilla extract
- 1 tsp cinnamon
- 2 cups tofu
- 1 egg white
- ¼ cup ground almonds
- ¼ cup brown rice flakes

Nutritional Value:

- Calories: 200
- Carbohydrates: 218.3 g
- Protein: 7.6 g
- Fat: 10.7 g

3. In a mini food processor, process the sunflower, pumpkin, and toasted sesame seeds until they form a powder. Transfer to a bowl and add the ground hazelnuts and mixed/apple pie spice. Mix well. Add the fig puree and enough cold water to form a dough.

4. Line the base of the baking tin with the dough, using your hands to flatten it. Bake for about 10 minutes until golden. Remove from the oven and set aside.

5. To make the filling, blend the apples and tofu with ½ scant cup of water until a thick paste forms. Transfer to a large mixing bowl.

6. In another bowl, whisk the egg white until stiff peaks form. Gently fold the beaten egg white into the apple mixture. Add the lemon juice, vanilla extract, cinnamon, and ground almonds. Mix gently.

209

For greasing:

- Soy margarine

7. Spoon the filling onto the pastry case/pie shell and sprinkle the brown rice flakes over the top.

8. Bake for 30 minutes or until set.

9. Allow the cheesecake to cool for 5 minutes, then remove it from the pan. Let it cool completely at room temperature, then chill in the refrigerator for several hours or overnight.

10. Serve the Apple & Tofu Cheesecake chilled.

6.

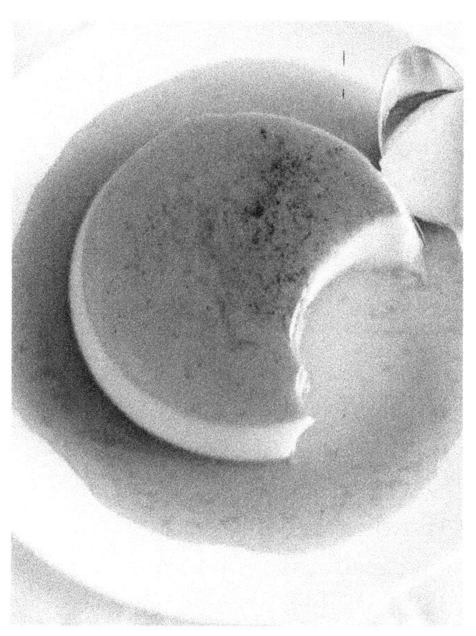

Crème Caramel

Prep Time   Cook Time   Servings

15 min   50 min   4

Method:

INGREDIENTS:

- Sunflower oil for greasing

- ¼ cup golden caster/superfine sugar, plus 2 tbsp

- 3 large eggs, beaten
- 1 scant cup soy milk
- ½ tsp vanilla extract

1. Grease a small saucepan with sunflower oil. Add 2 tablespoons of water to the saucepan, then add the sugar. Heat gently over low heat until the sugar has dissolved. Increase the heat to medium-high and bring it to a boil without stirring. Cook for 3 minutes until the syrup turns a deep golden color and becomes syrupy. Remove from heat and stir in 2 teaspoons of boiling water.

2. Preheat the oven to 160°C/325°F/Gas 3. Grease a 2

211

For serving:

- Soy cream

Nutritional Value:

- Calories: 182

- Carbohydrates: 21.5 g

- Protein: 9.1 g

- Fat: 6.3 g

½-cup ovenproof dish with sunflower oil. Pour the sugar syrup into the dish, tilting it to ensure the bottom is completely covered.

3. In a bowl, beat the eggs with the soy milk. Add the sugar and vanilla extract, and beat again until thoroughly combined. Strain the mixture into the greased ovenproof dish through a sieve/fine-mesh strainer. Place the dish in a roasting pan and pour enough water into the roasting pan to come halfway up the sides of the ovenproof dish.

4. Bake for 50 minutes or until the custard is set. Remove the dish from the oven and let it cool for 30 minutes. Once cooled, carefully turn out the crème caramel onto a serving dish. Chill in the refrigerator for 1 hour before serving.

5. Serve the Crème Caramel chilled, optionally topped with soy cream.

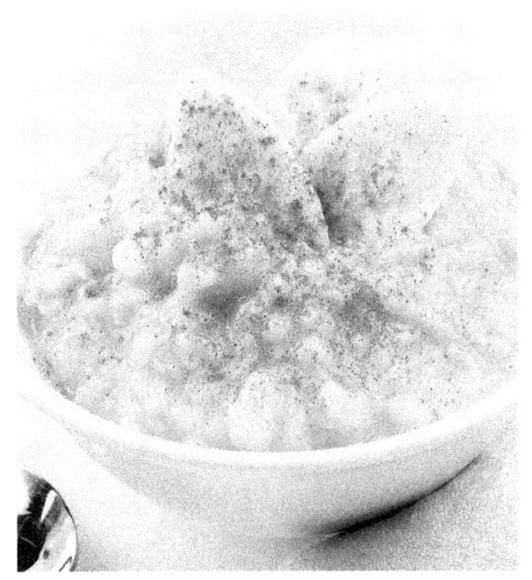

Banana & Rice Pudding

Prep Time	Cook Time	Servings
10 min	1½-2 hrs	5

INGREDIENTS:

- Zest of 1 lemon
- 2 mashed bananas
- 3 cups soy milk
- 1 tsp vanilla extract
- 1 tsp ground nutmeg
- 1 scant cup short-grain rice

Method:

1. Preheat the oven to 180°C/350°F/Gas 4. Mix the mashed bananas, rice, soy milk, vanilla extract, and lemon zest in a bowl until thoroughly combined.

2. Transfer the mixture to a 7-scant cup ovenproof dish. Using a fine sieve/strainer, sprinkle the ground nutmeg over the top.

3. Bake in the preheated oven for 1 ½-2 hours until the pudding is firm and the rice is cooked.

213

For serving:

- Sugar-free jam

Nutritional Value:

- Calories: 227
- Carbohydrates:

41.5 g

- Protein: 9.1 g
- Fat: 3.2 g
-

4. Serve the banana and rice pudding hot, and if desired, top with sugar-free jam.

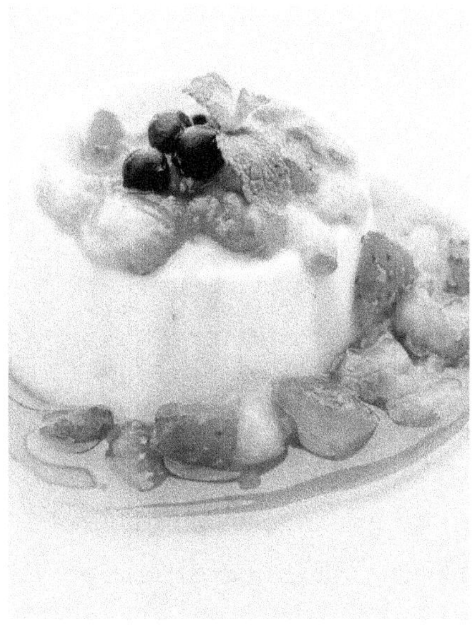

INGREDIENTS:

- ½ cup pitted prunes

(soaked overnight)

- 2 cups silken tofu

- 2 tbsp maple syrup

Prune & Tofu Dessert

Prep Time   Cook Time   Servings

15min   15 min   4

Method:

1. Place the prunes in a bowl and cover them with water. Let them soak for at least 12 hours or overnight. Drain the prunes and transfer them to a saucepan. Add enough water to cover the prunes and boil over medium heat. Reduce the heat to a simmer and cook for 10-15 minutes until the prunes are very tender. Drain the prunes, reserving the cooking liquid.

215

For serving:

- Blueberries or strawberries

Nutritional Value:

- Calories: 127
- Carbohydrates: 8.4 g
- Protein: 10.2 g
- Fat: 5.7 g

2. Combine the cooked prunes, silken tofu, and maple syrup in a blender or food processor. While blending, gradually add the reserved cooking liquid until thick and smooth puree forms.

3. Transfer the mixture to a bowl and refrigerate for 15 minutes to chill. Serve the prune and tofu dessert sprinkled with blueberries or strawberries.

4. Note: You can adjust the sweetness by adding more or less maple syrup according to your preference.

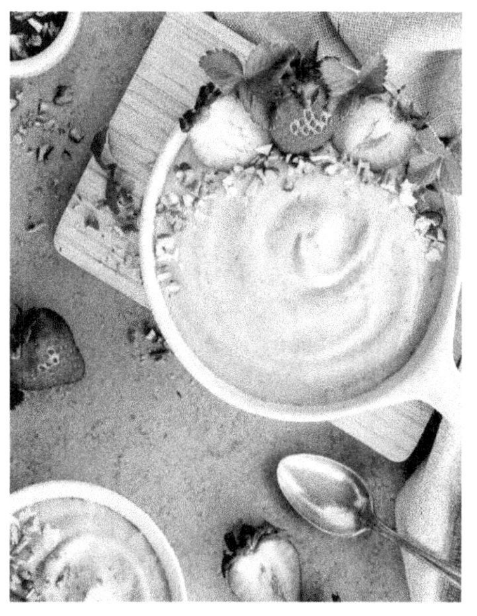

Tofu Strawberry Dessert

Prep Time	Cook Time	Servings
15min	15 min	4

INGREDIENTS:

- 2 tbsp port wine
- 2 cups silken tofu
- 3 tbsp clear honey
- 2 tsp vanilla extract
- 15 hulled & halved

vertically strawberries

- ½ heaped cup flaked/

sliced almonds

Method:

1. In a bowl, combine the strawberries and port wine. Gently mix them and let them stand for 1 hour to marinate. After marinating, drain the strawberries and set them aside.

2. In another bowl, mash the silken tofu well with a fork. Add the honey and vanilla extract to the tofu, and mix until well combined.

Nutritional Value:

- Calories: 230

- Carbohydrates: 14.9 g

- Protein: 12.2 g

- Fat: 10.8 g

3. To serve, spoon the tofu mixture into individual serving dishes. Top with the marinated strawberries and sprinkle with flaked or sliced almonds.

4. Note: You can adjust the sweetness by adding more or less honey according to your taste preference.

5.

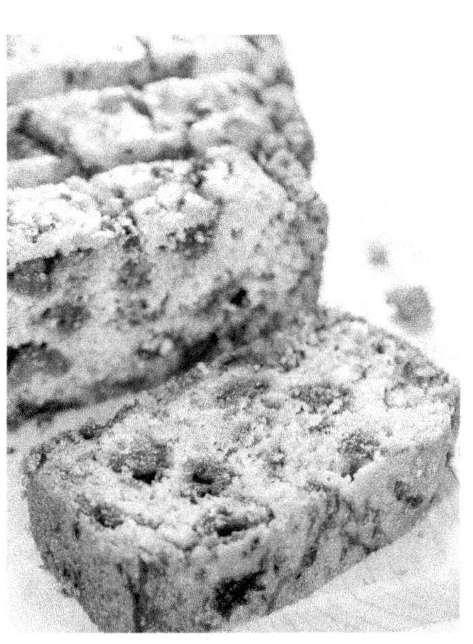

Banana & Raspberry Bread

  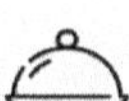

Prep Time	Cook Time	Servings
15min	1 hr	10

INGREDIENTS:

- 1 cup mashed ripe bananas
- ½ cup soy milk
- 1/4 cup vegetable oil
- ½ cup roughly chopped roasted hazelnuts
- 2 beaten eggs
- ½ cup soft light brown sugar
- 1 ¾ cups self-rising flour

Method:

1. Preheat the oven to 350°F/Gas 4 and lightly grease an 8 ½ x 4 ¼ inch loaf pan with sunflower oil.

2. In a large mixing bowl, beat the mashed bananas, vegetable oil, eggs, brown sugar, and soy milk until well combined.

3. Sift the self-rising flour, plain flour, and ground cinnamon into the banana mixture. Fold the dry

219

- ⅔ cup scant plain/all-purpose flour

- 1 tsp ground cinnamon
- ½ cup dried banana, chopped

- 1 cup raspberries

For serving:

- Sunflower oil
- Soy cream cheese
- Clear honey

Nutritional Value:

- Calories: 262
- Carbohydrates: 35.2 g
- Protein: 5.9 g
- Fat: 10.8 g

ingredients into the wet ingredients until just combined.

4. Add the chopped hazelnuts, dried banana, and raspberries to the batter. Gently fold them in, being careful not to over-mix.

5. Spoon the batter into the prepared loaf pan and smooth the top with a spatula.

6. Bake for approximately 1 hour until the bread is golden and a skewer inserted into the middle comes clean.

7. Remove the bread from the oven and let it cool in the pan for 5 minutes. Then, transfer it to a wire rack to cool completely.

8. Once cooled, slice the banana and raspberry bread and serve with soy cream cheese and a drizzle of clear honey.

6.

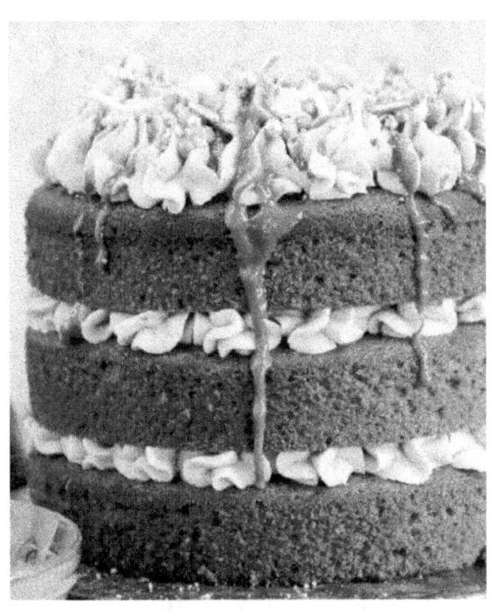

Ginger Cake

  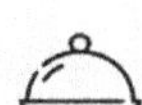

Prep Time   Cook Time   Servings

15min   1 hr   10

INGREDIENTS:

- 1/2 cup sunflower margarine
- ½ cup golden syrup
- ½ cup treacle
- 2 tsp ground ginger
- ½ tsp mixed spice
- ½ tsp baking powder
- 2 beaten eggs
- sugar

Method:

1. Preheat the oven to 325°F/Gas 3 and grease an 8-in loose-bottomed cake pan with sunflower oil.

2. In a saucepan over medium heat, melt the sunflower margarine and sugar together. Gradually pour in the golden syrup and treacle, and stir in the ground ginger and mixed spice.

3. Sift the maize meal, potato flour, rice flour, and baking powder into a large mixing bowl. Mix them,

221

- ½ cup milk
- ⅓ cup maize meal
- ½ heaped cup potato

flour

- ½ heaped cup rice flour
- ⅓ heaped cup dark

muscovado

For greasing:

- Sunflower oil

Nutritional Value:

- Calories: 278
- Carbohydrates: 36.6 g
- Protein: 5 g
- Fat: 12.4 g

create a well in the center and pour in the syrup mixture. Using a wooden spoon, beat until the batter is smooth.

4. In a separate bowl, beat the eggs and milk together. Gradually pour this mixture into the cake batter, beating continuously to keep the mixture smooth.

5. Pour the cake batter into the prepared cake pan and bake for approximately 1 hour, or until the cake is cooked and a skewer inserted into the center comes clean.

6. Remove the cake from the oven and let it cool in the pan for 5 minutes. Then, turn it onto a wire rack and let it cool completely before serving.

5.

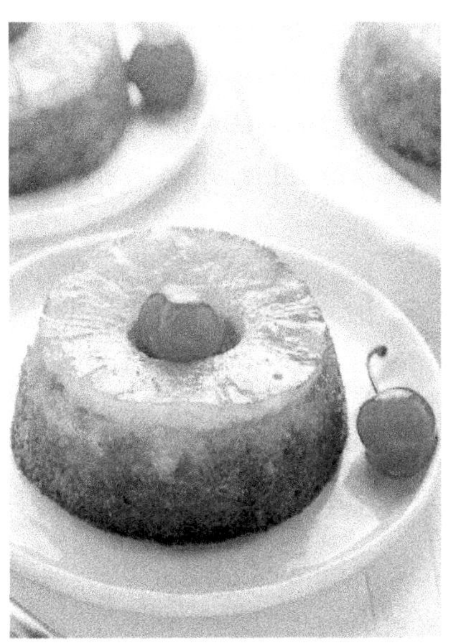

Pineapple Cake

  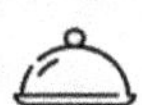

Prep Time	Cook Time	Servings
15min	40 min	10

Method:

INGREDIENTS:

- ⅓ heaped cup (100 g) prunes, pitted & finely chopped prunes
- 4 tbsp dried figs
- 4 beaten eggs
- ⅔ heaped cup ground almonds

1. Preheat the oven to 350°F/Gas 4 and grease an 8-in loose-bottomed baking pan with sunflower oil.

2. In a saucepan, mix together the chopped prunes, dried figs, and just under ⅔ cup of water. Heat the mixture over medium heat until it reaches boiling point, then lower the heat to a gentle level and let it simmer for about 5 minutes or until the water has been soaked up and the fruits have turned soft. Allow the mixture to cool for a period of 10 minutes.

- 1 tsp baking soda
- ½ tsp baking powder
- 6 tbsp brown rice flour
- ⅔ cup finely chopped

pumpkin seeds

- 2 ¾ cups pineapple,

peeled, cored, & chopped

into ½ in pieces

- 4 tbsp raisins

For greasing:

- Sunflower oil

Nutritional Value:

- Calories: 251

- Carbohydrates: 33.3 g

- Protein: 7.6 g

- Fat: 9.8 g

3. In a mixing bowl, stir the chopped pineapple, raisins, and cooked fruit mixture.

4. Fold the beaten eggs into the fruit mixture in a separate clean bowl. Sift the ground almonds, baking soda, baking powder, and brown rice flour into the mixture. Add the finely chopped pumpkin seeds and fold everything together until well combined.

5. Pour the cake batter into the prepared baking pan and bake for 40 minutes, or until golden and a skewer inserted into the center comes out clean.

6. Remove the cake from the oven and let it cool in the pan for 5 minutes. Then, transfer it onto a wire rack and allow it to cool completely before serving.

7.

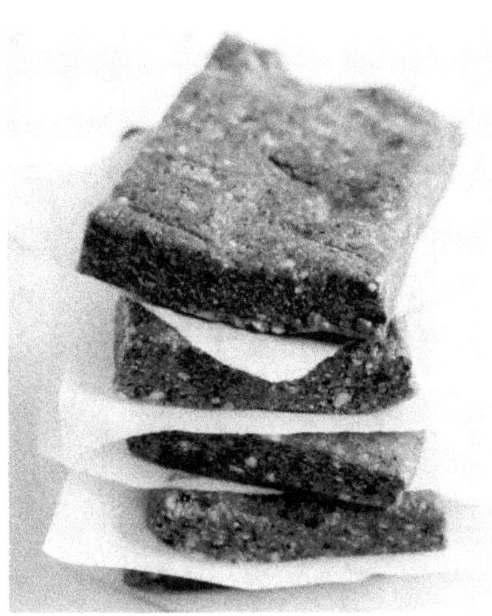

INGREDIENTS:

- ⅔ cup flaxseeds
- 1 cup date syrup
- ⅓ cup sesame seeds
- ½ cup sunflower seeds
- ½ cup pumpkin seeds
- ¾ cup soy protein

isolate or soy protein

powder

- 6 cups puffed rice
- 2 tsp mixed/apple

pie spice

Phyto Fix Bars

Prep Time	Cook Time	Servings
10 min	20 min	10

Method:

7. Preheat the oven to 350°F/Gas 4 and grease a 12 x 8 x 1-inch baking pan with sunflower oil.

8. In a large mixing bowl, combine the sesame seeds, flaxseeds, sunflower seeds, pumpkin seeds, dried vine fruits, dried apricots, soy protein isolate or soy protein powder, puffed rice, mixed/apple pie spice, and ground ginger (if using). Mix well.

9. Pour the date syrup, ginger or brown rice malt, and soy milk. Mix

- 2 tsp ground ginger
(optional)

- 1 ¾ cups ginger
syrup or brown rice
malt

- ⅔ scant cup soy milk
- ⅓ scant cup unsulphured
dried apricots, chopped

- ¾ heaped cup dried vine
fruits, such as raisins,
sultanas/golden raisins,
or currants

For greasing:

- Sunflower oil

Nutritional Value:

- Calories: 359

thoroughly until all the ingredients are well combined and evenly coated.

10. Spoon the mixture into the greased baking pan and use a palette knife/metal spatula or the back of a spoon to smooth the surface.

11. Bake for 20 minutes or until golden. Remove from the oven and let it cool for 5 minutes.

12. Cut the mixture into 8 bars while it is still warm. Allow the bars to cool completely before serving.

13.

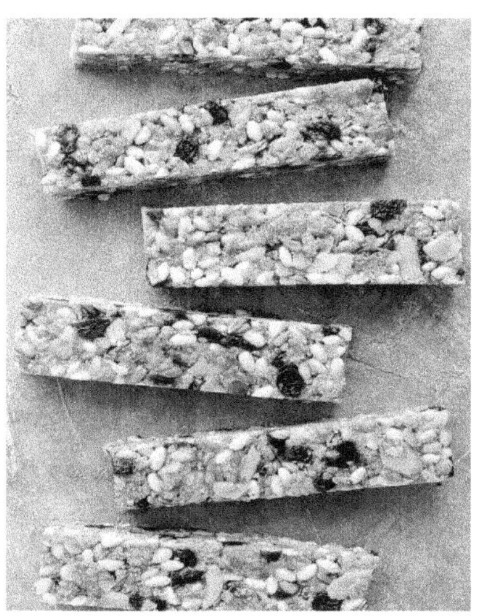

Chewy Fruit Bars

Prep Time   Cook Time   Servings

10 min 5 min(Refg T 3 hr) 10

INGREDIENTS:

- ½ scant cup orange

juice

- 1 tsp grated orange zest
- ⅓ cup almonds, chopped
- ½ cup plus extra

for sprinkling desiccated/

dried shredded coconut

- 3 cups puffed rice
- 1 cup ground almonds

Method:

1. Preheat the oven to 350°F/Gas 4 and line a baking sheet with foil.

2. Combine the orange juice, chopped apricots, and zest in a medium-sized saucepan. Bring to a boil over medium heat, then reduce the heat to low, and let it simmer for 5 minutes or until the liquid has been absorbed and the apricots are soft. Transfer the mixture to a large mixing bowl.

3. Place the chopped almonds and coconut on separate baking sheets.

227

- 4 tbsp clear honey
- ½ heaped cup

unsulphured dried

chopped apricots

- 1 ¾ oz/½ scant cup
- chopped dried fruit,

such as raisins, apples,

or peach

- Toasted flaked/sliced
- almonds for sprinkling

Nutritional Value:

- Calories: 174
- Carbohydrates: 17 g
- Protein: 5.6 g
- Fat: 9.2 g

Bake the almonds for 3-4 minutes until heated, and the coconut for 1 minute or until lightly golden.

4. Add the puffed rice, ground almonds, coconut, almonds, honey, and dried fruit to the apricot mixture. Stir well to combine.

5. Shape the mixture into a large ball and flatten it using your hands. Transfer the mixture to the foil-lined baking sheet and press it evenly to the edges of the pan.

6. Sprinkle the mixture with coconut and the toasted flaked/sliced almonds. Cut the mixture into 12 bars. Chill the bars in the refrigerator for about 3 hours to set.

7. Store the bars in a sealed container in the refrigerator and consume them within 1 week.

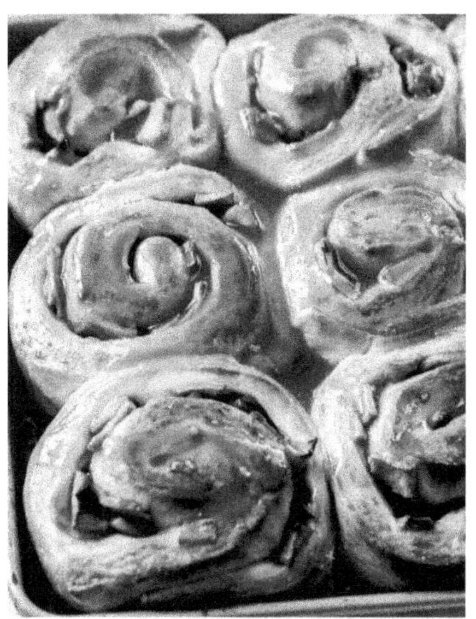

Apple Walnuut Coffee Rolls

Prep Time 20 min

Cook Time 55 min

Servings 10

INGREDIENTS:

- ¾ cup butter
- 1 cup soy milk
- ½ tsp cinnamon
- ½ cup chopped walnuts
- 2 ¾ oz soft light brown

sugar

- 3 cups tart green apples,
- peeled, cored, & diced
- 3 ¼ cups self-rising

flour, plus extra for dusting

Method:

1. Cut 1 oz of the butter into cubes and chill in the refrigerator.

2. Heat the remaining butter in a frying pan over medium heat until melted. Add the apples and walnuts and cook, stirring occasionally, for 5 minutes or until the apples soften. Add the cinnamon and sugar and cook, stirring frequently, for 6 minutes, until the sugar caramelizes. Remove from heat and let it cool for 5 minutes.

229

For the frosting:

- 1 tsp coffee granules

- ⅔ scant cup icing/

confectioners' sugar

Nutritional Value:

- Calories: 368

- Carbohydrates: 43.9 g

- Protein: 6.2 g

- Fat: 18.6 g

3. Pass the flour through a sieve into a spacious mixing bowl and incorporate the chilled butter. Use your fingertips to work the butter into the flour until the mixture takes on the appearance of fine breadcrumbs. Create a hollow space in the middle and pour in the soy milk. Mix the soy milk into the mixture using a round-bladed knife in a cutting action to form a stiff dough. Press the dough into a ball with your hands, adding more flour if the dough is sticky. Cover with cling film/plastic wrap and chill in the refrigerator for 30 minutes.

4. Preheat the oven to 400°F/Gas 6 and line a baking sheet with parchment. Place the dough on a lightly floured surface and press it into an 8 x 12-inch rectangle. Spread the apple mixture over the dough, then roll up the dough from the long side to enclose the

230

filling. Place the roll seam-side on a chopping board and cut it into 8 pieces. Place this cut-side on the baking sheet and bake for 20 minutes or until golden brown. Remove from the sheet and let them cool on a wire rack.

8. To make the frosting, put the coffee granules in a small bowl and add 1 tablespoon of hot water. Mix well, then quickly stir in the icing/confectioners' sugar until the mixture is smooth. Drizzle the frosting over the rolls with a spoon and let it set for 30 minutes. Serve and enjoy!

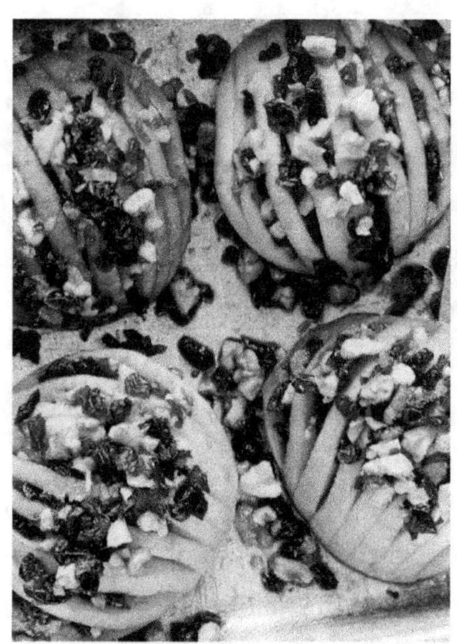

Apple stuffed with Nuts and Sultanas

Prep Time	Cook Time	Servings
10min	40 min	4

Method:

INGREDIENTS:

- 2 tbsp melted butter

or ghee

- 2 tbsp sultanas or dried

cranberries

- A pinch of cinnamon
- 2 tbsp roughly chopped

nuts of your choice

- 4 large apples, ideally

Bramley or Granny

Smith, cored

1. Preheat the oven to 400°F/Gas 6. Mix the melted butter, chopped nuts, sultanas, and cinnamon in a bowl.

2. Stand the apples upright in a baking dish, ensuring they remain stable. Stuff each apple with the nut mixture using a spoon or your fingers. Spread any leftover butter onto the apples.

3. Bake for 20-40 minutes until the apples are tender, cooked, and

232

- For serving: yogurt (optional)

Nutritional Value:

- Calories: 183

- Carbohydrates: 22.3 g

- Protein: 1.3 g

- Fat: 10 g

slightly caramelized. The exact cooking time will depend on the type of apple used.

4. Serve the apples warm on their own or with a dollop of yogurt if desired.

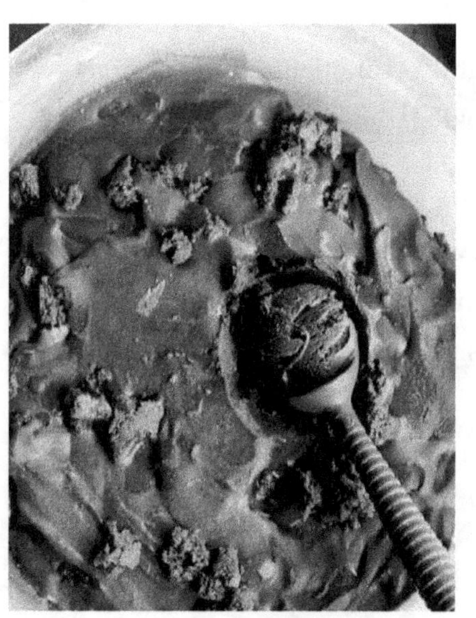

Banana, Ruspberryand chocolate ice Cream

Prep Time	Cook Time	Servings
5 min	4 hr(Refg. T)	1

INGREDIENTS:

Banana Flavor:

- 2 bananas
- 4 tbsp unsweetened

milk of your choice

- ½ tsp vanilla extract

(optional)

- Honey or maple
- syrup to sweeten

(optional)

Method:

1. Peel the bananas, cut them into 4 portions, and place them in a bag in the freezer for 4 hours (or overnight) until they are frozen.

2. For each flavor option, blend or pulse all the ingredients together in a food processor until smooth. If needed, scrape the sides of the blender and pulse again. Adjust the consistency by adding extra

Raspberry Flavor:

- 1 banana
- 1 cup froze

raspberries

- 4 tbsp unsweetened milk

of your choice

- Honey or maple syrup to

sweeten (optional)

milk, and sweeten with honey or maple syrup, if desired.

3. Scoop the ice cream into a bowl and enjoy immediately.

Chocolate Flavor:

- 1 banana
- 4 tbsp unsweetened milk of your choice
- 1 ½ tbsp 100% raw unsweetened cacao powder
- 1 tbsp clear honey or maple syrup

Nutritional Value:

- Calories: 339
- Carbohydrates: 63.2 g
- Protein: 6.5 g

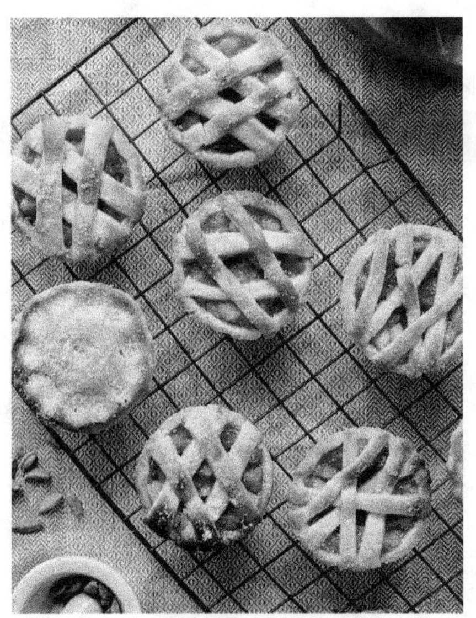

INGREDIENTS:

For the pastry:

- 1 cup walnuts
- 1 large egg
- 2 tsp coconut flour
- ¼ tsp sea salt

Cinnamon Apple
Tart

Prep Time	Cook Time	Servings
25 min	45-60 min	4

Method:

1. Preheat the oven to 400°F/Gas 6.

2. To make the pastry crust, pulse the walnuts in a food processor until they resemble coarse gravel. Transfer the walnut mixture to a large bowl and add pastry ingredients. Mix well until a ball of dough forms.

3. Line a 9-in tart tin with parchment paper. Using wet fingers, press the pastry into the bottom and around the sides of the tin.

236

For the filling:

- 1 ½ lb apples, peeled, cored, & sliced
- 1 tbsp lemon juice
- 1 tbsp corn flour
- 1 tbsp clear honey
- 1 tbsp cinnamon

Nutritional Value:

- Calories: 320

- Carbohydrates: 25.7 g

- Protein: 7.7 g

- Fat: 20.5 g

4. In a large bowl, combine all the filling ingredients and toss to coat the apple slices.

5. Arrange the apple slices in a fan shape on top of the pastry, creating a small circle at the center and a wider circle around it.

6. Bake for 45-60 minutes until the apples are cooked, and the pastry is golden brown.

7. Serve the cinnamon apple tart warm or cold.

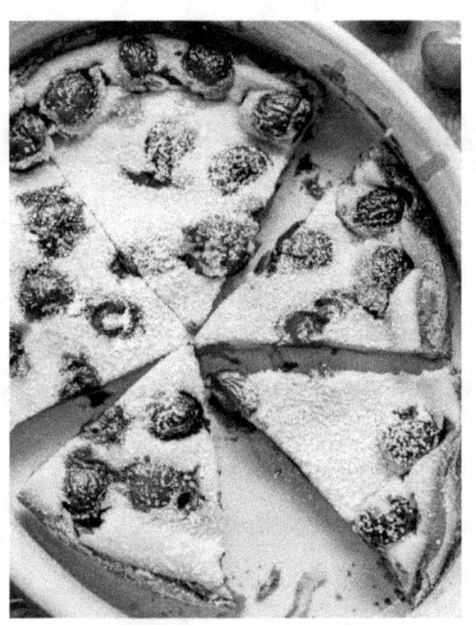

Fruit Clafoutis

Prep Time	Cook Time	Servings
5 min	45 min	4

INGREDIENTS:

- 2 ¾ cups frozen

or fresh fruits

- 4 eggs
- 1 cup gluten-free flour
- 1 cup whole milk

or unsweetened milk

of your choice

- ¾ cup sugar

Method:

8. Preheat the oven to 400°F/Gas 6. Line a 9-in round oven tin with parchment paper. Arrange the fruits evenly in the tin.

9. Whisk together the eggs, gluten-free flour, milk, and sugar in a bowl until smooth.

10. Pour the egg mixture over the fruits in the tin.

11. Bake for 40-45 minutes until the clafoutis is cooked through and golden on top.

238

For the Serving:

- Yogurt (optional)

Nutritional Value:

- Calories: 392
- Carbohydrates: 73 g
- Protein: 11.9 g
- Fat: 5.8 g

12. Serve the fruit clafoutis warm or cold. Optionally, serve with a dollop of yogurt.

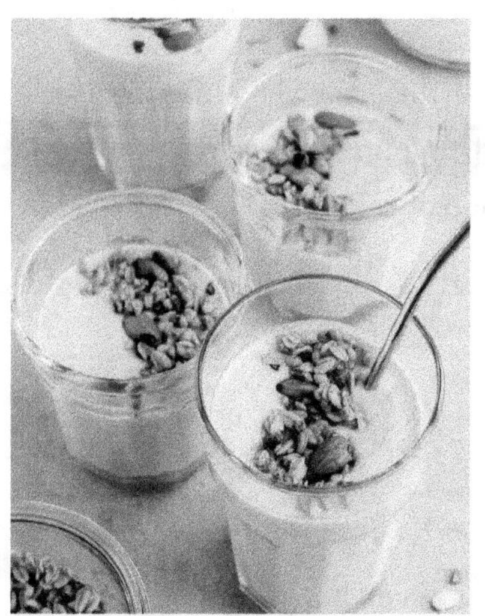

INGREDIENTS:

- 1 ¼ tbsp ground
- turmeric
- 2 tsp ground ginger
- 2 tsp cinnamon
- 1 ¼ tbsp clear honey
- 1 liter unsweetened
- milk of your choice

Nutritional Value:

- Calories: 155
- Carbohydrates: 18.7 g
- Protein: 9.5 g
- Fat: 4.6 g

Golden Milk

Prep Time	Cook Time	Servings
2 min	5 min	4

Method:

1. Place all the ingredients in a food processor and blend until well combined.

2. Pour the mixture into a small pan and heat over medium heat for 3-5 minutes until hot but not boiling.

3. Serve the golden milk immediately.

4.

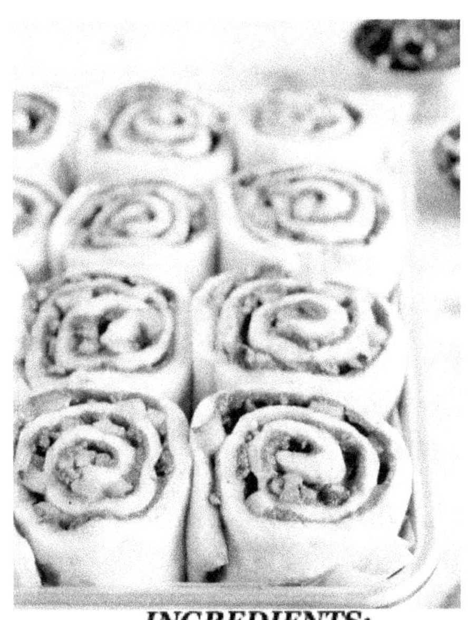

Apple Bread Rolls

Prep Time	Cook Time	Servings
5 min	45 min	4

INGREDIENTS:

- 2 eggs
- 1 cup tofu
- 1 cup grated apple
- ½ tsp cream of tartar
- ¼ tsp tartaric acid
- 1 tbsp olive oil
- ½ scant cup potato flour
- ½ scant cup rice flour
- ½ heaped cup soy flour

Method:

1. Preheat the oven to 220°C/425°F/Gas 7 and grease a 12-hole muffin pan with soy margarine.

2. Whisk together the tofu, grated apple, soy milk, and eggs in a bowl until smooth. Set aside.

3. In a large mixing bowl, sift the potato flour, rice flour, soy flour, cornmeal, baking soda, cream of tartar, and tartaric acid. Add the olive oil and sugar, and mix well.

241

- ½ scant cup cornmeal
- ⅔ scant cup unsweetened soy milk
- 1 tsp baking soda
- 1 tsp Golden caster/ superfine sugar

For Greasing:

- Soy margarine

Nutritional Value:

- Calories: 203
- Carbohydrates: 27.2 g
- Protein: 9 g
- Fat: 6.4 g

4. Fold the tofu mixture into the dry ingredients, careful not to over-mix. Make sure the batter is well combined but still light.

5. Spoon the batter into the greased muffin pan, filling each hole about three-quarters full.

6. Bake in the preheated oven for 12-15 minutes or until golden and a toothpick inserted into the center comes out clean.

7. Remove from the oven and let the rolls cool in the pan for 5 minutes. Then transfer them to a wire rack to cool completely.

8. Serve the apple bread rolls warm with sweet or savory dishes

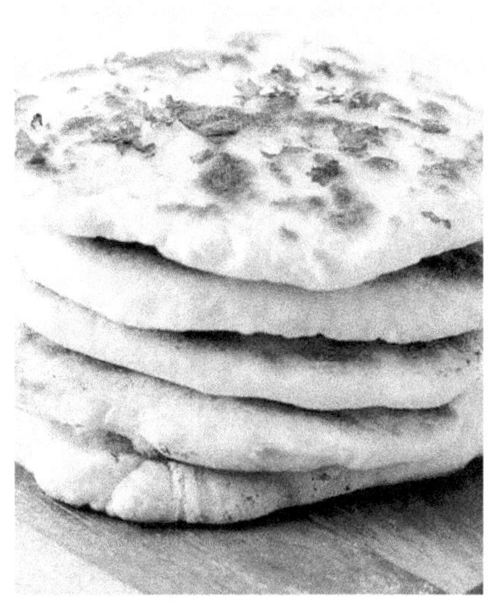

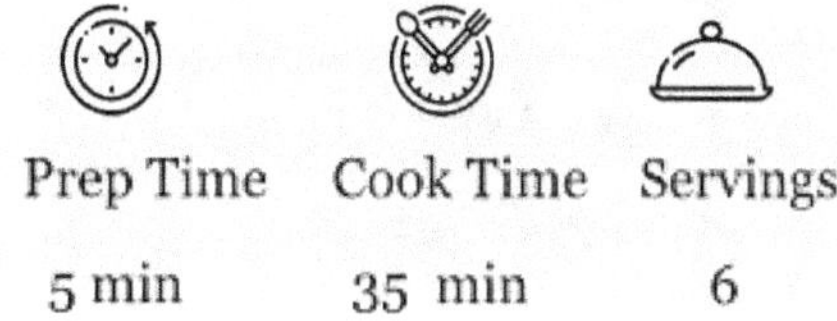

Prep Time	Cook Time	Servings
5 min	35 min	6

INGREDIENTS:

- 1 egg
- 1 cup tofu
- 1 tbsp soy oil
- ¾ heaped cup rice flour
- ½ scant cup maize flour
- 1 tbsp soy flour
- 1 tsp cream of tartar
- ½ tsp tartaric acid

Method:

1. Preheat the oven to 425°F/Gas 7 and line a 10-inch square baking sheet with parchment.

2. Combine the tofu, egg, and soy milk in a blender or food processor. Blend until smooth.

3. In a bowl, sift the rice flour, maize flour, soy flour, baking soda, cream of tartar, tartaric acid, and sugar. Stir in the soy oil and mix well.

243

- ⅔ scant cup unsweetened

soy milk

- 1 tsp baking soda
- 1 tsp Golden caster/
- superfine sugar

Nutritional Value:

- Calories: 217
- Carbohydrates: 29 g
- Protein: 8.9 g
- Fat: 7.1 g

4. Fold the tofu mixture into the dry ingredients, careful not to over mix. The dough should be well combined but not heavy.

5. Spoon the dough onto the prepared baking sheet and spread it evenly using a palette knife, metal spatula, or the back of a spoon.

6. Bake in the oven for 35 minutes or until the flatbread is lightly golden.

7. Remove from the oven and let it cool for 5 minutes. Transfer to a wire rack to cool completely.

8. Serve the flatbread warm.

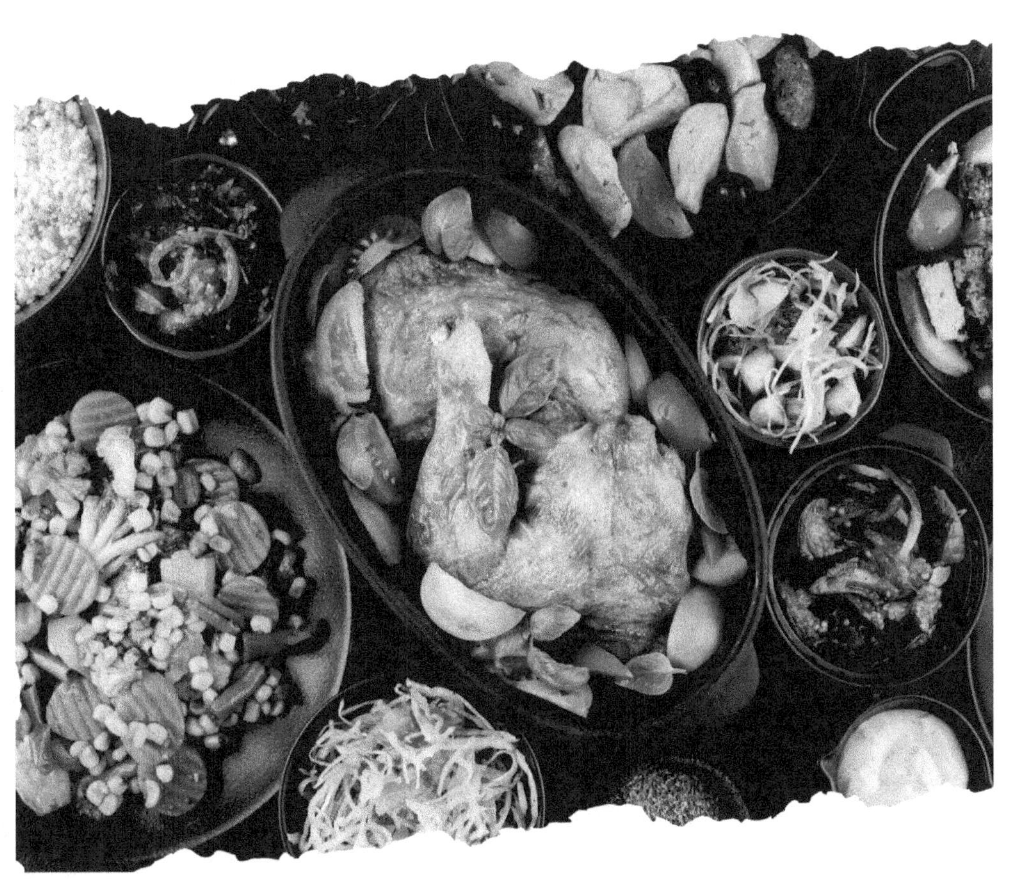

Dinner Recipes

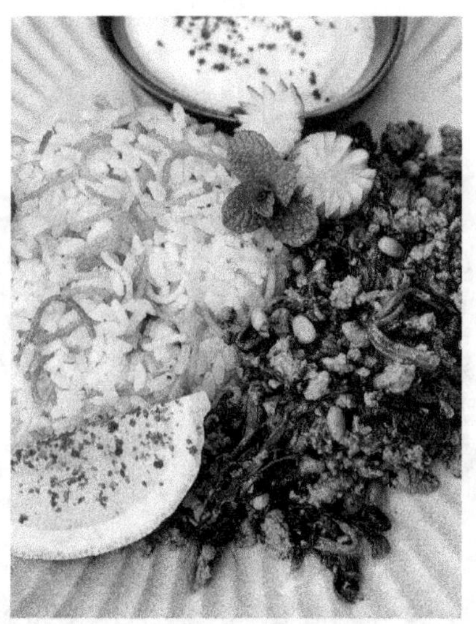

Beef, Spinach & Spices with Rice

Prep Time	Cook Time	Servings
5 min	25 min	6

INGREDIENTS:

- 2 cups basmati rice
- 3 tsp butter or ghee
- 1 large onion, finely chopped
- 1 lb minced beef
- 1 tbsp Lebanese 7 spice
- 1 tbsp allspice
- 3 cups baby spinach
- Juice of 1 lemon
- 1 tbsp roasted pine nuts

Method:

1. Cook the basmati rice according to the packet instructions.

2. Heat the butter or ghee over medium heat in a large frying pan. Add the chopped onion and cook, stirring, for about 5 minutes until translucent.

3. Increase the heat to high and add the minced beef to the pan. Break the beef into small pieces using two wooden spoons and cook for about 5 minutes until browned.

For garnish:

- Coriander

Nutritional Value:

- Calories: 441

- Carbohydrates: 44.2 g

- Protein: 24.3 g

- Fat: 18.3 g

4. Add the Lebanese 7 spice and allspice to the pan, and mix well with the meat. Reduce the heat to low.

5. Add half of the baby spinach to the pan and stir until wilted. Then, add the remaining spinach and mix well. Simmer for 8-10 minutes.

6. Turn off the heat and drizzle the lemon juice over the beef and spinach mixture, stirring to combine.

7. Divide the cooked basmati rice among the serving plates. Top with the beef and spinach mixture. Sprinkle roasted pine nuts over the dish and garnish with coriander.

8. Serve the Beef, Spinach and Spices with Rice immediately.

Lamb Stew

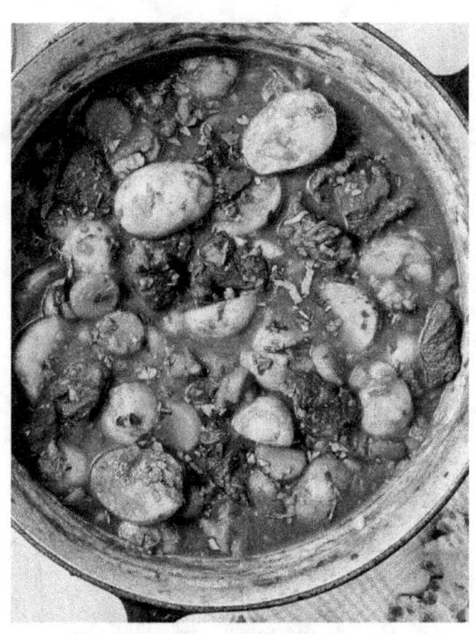

Prep Time	Cook Time	Servings
20 min	90 min	4

INGREDIENTS:

- 2 tbsp olive oil
- 1 tbsp ras el hanout
- 1 tsp ground coriander
- 1 large onion, finely chopped

- 2 garlic cloves, finely chopped

- 2 cups butternut squash, diced

Method:

1. Heat the olive oil in a flameproof casserole dish. Add the chopped onion and cook for 5 minutes until softened.

2. Add the chopped garlic and spices (ras el hanout and ground coriander) to the casserole dish and cook for another 2 minutes, stirring well.

3. Add the diced lamb, butternut squash, and soft dried apricots to the dish. Pour in the chopped

- 1 cup soft dried apricots
- 3 ¼ cups can chopped

tomatoes

- 2 cups bone broth
- Sea salt and freshly

ground black pepper

- Zest of 1 lemon
- 1 1/3 lb leg of lamb,

diced into ¾-in

pieces, excess fat trimmed

For serving:

- Chopped coriander leaves
- Quinoa and yogurt

Nutritional Value:

- Calories: 517
- Carbohydrates: 25.2 g
- Protein: 34.4 g
- Fat: 30 g

tomatoes and bone broth. Season well with salt and pepper.

4. Heat the mixture until it reaches a boiling point, then lower the temperature to a gentle simmer. Place a lid on the casserole dish and allow it to cook slowly for approximately 1 hour, occasionally stirring.

5. Remove the lid and continue cooking for 30 minutes to allow the flavors to develop.

6. Check the seasoning and adjust if needed. Sprinkle the lemon zest and chopped coriander over the tagine.

7. Serve the Lamb Tagine in warm bowls, accompanied by quinoa and yogurt.

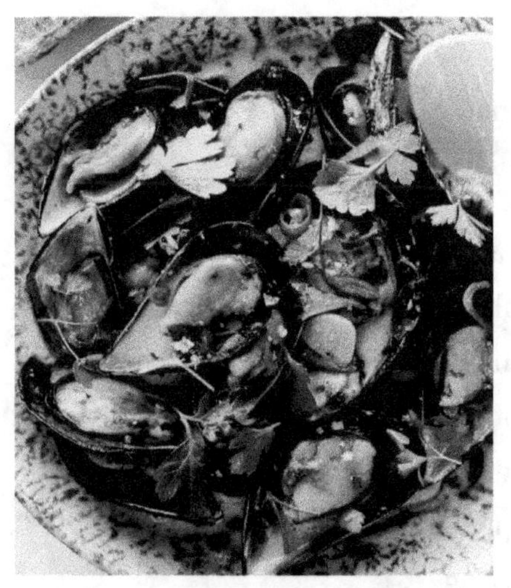

Mussels in White Wine

Prep Time   Cook Time   Servings

10 min   15 min   5

INGREDIENTS:

- 1 tbsp butter or ghee
- 2 shallots, thinly sliced
- 2 garlic cloves, thinly sliced
- 1 ½ cups dry white wine
- 4 ½ lb cleaned mussels

Method:

8. Melt the butter or ghee over medium heat in a large pot with a lid. Once the butter begins to foam, add the shallots and garlic. Cook until softened, approximately 5 minutes.

9. Pour in the white wine and add the mussels. Give them a good stir and cover the pot with the lid.

10. After a few minutes, turn and mix the mussels to facilitate an easy opening. Replace the lid and cook for a few more minutes until all

250

the mussels have opened. Discard any mussels that remain closed.

11. Sprinkle with finely chopped parsley and serve immediately with potato wedges on the side.

For garnish:

- 1 tbsp finely chopped

flat-leaf parsley

Nutritional Value:

- Calories: 385
- Carbohydrates: 14 g
- Protein: 47.1 g
- Fat: 13.3 g

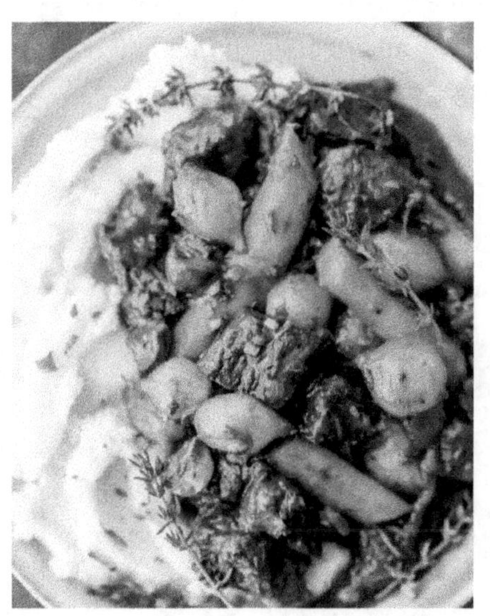

Beef Bourguignon

Prep Time	Cook Time	Servings
15 min	2 hr. 30 min	6

INGREDIENTS:

- 4 tbsp olive oil
- 2 tbsp corn flour
- 2 tsp butter or ghee
- ¾ cup bone broth
- 2 large bay leaves
- 1 onion, finely chopped
- 2 garlic cloves, crushed
-

Method:

1. Heat a large flameproof casserole dish over low heat, add 2 tablespoons of olive oil, and cook the onion until softened for about 5 minutes. Add the garlic and cook for another minute. Add the remaining olive oil and fry the beef until browned.

- 4 carrots, roughly

chopped

- 2 tbsp tomato purée
- 3 sprigs thyme
- Sea salt & freshly

ground black pepper

- 2 ¾ cups halved small

chestnut mushrooms

- 2 lb braising beef, fat

or sinew trimmed, cut

into 1 ½ - 2 inch chunks

Nutritional Value:

- Calories: 555

- Carbohydrates: 12.2 g

- Protein: 42.8 g

- Fat: 37 g

2. Add the carrots, tomato purée, bone broth, and herbs. Season and bring to a simmer. Stir, cover with a lid, and cook for about 1 ½ hours on low heat.

3. In the meantime, heat a large frying pan over medium heat. Melt the butter or ghee, add the mushrooms, and cook until golden. Set aside. Place the corn flour and 2 tablespoons of water in a bowl and mix until smooth.

4. Stir in the corn flour mixture, add the mushrooms, and cook for another 45 minutes until the beef is tender and the sauce has thickened. Remove the thyme sprigs and serve.

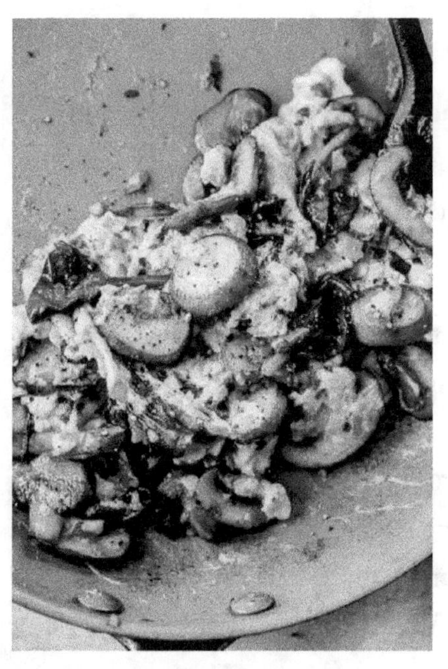

Bacon, Mushroom and Egg Cauliflower Bowl

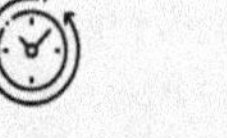  

Prep Time	Cook Time	Servings
15 min	20 min	8

INGREDIENTS:

- 8 eggs
- 4 tbsp olive oil
- 1 thinly sliced large onion
- 4 ½ cups grated cauliflower
- 1 tbsp thyme leaves
- 2 tbsp tamari soy sauce

Method:

1. Heat a frying pan over medium heat and cook the bacon until desired tenderness. Set aside.

2. Add 1 tablespoon of olive oil to the pan and sauté the onion for a few minutes. Add another tablespoon of olive oil, the mushrooms, and tamari soy sauce. Cook until the mushrooms are tender. Add the

- 8 slices preservative-free bacon

- 4 cups finely chopped mushrooms

Nutritional Value:

- Calories: 227
- Carbohydrates: 4.1 g
- Protein: 16.2 g
- Fat: 16 g

thyme leaves and mix well. Remove from heat and set aside.

3. Add the remaining olive oil to the same pan and cook the grated cauliflower for 5-7 minutes, stirring frequently. Return the cooked mushrooms to the pan and mix them with the cauliflower.

4. Prepare the eggs as desired: poached, scrambled, or fried.

5. Divide the cauliflower mixture among serving plates and top with the cooked eggs and bacon.

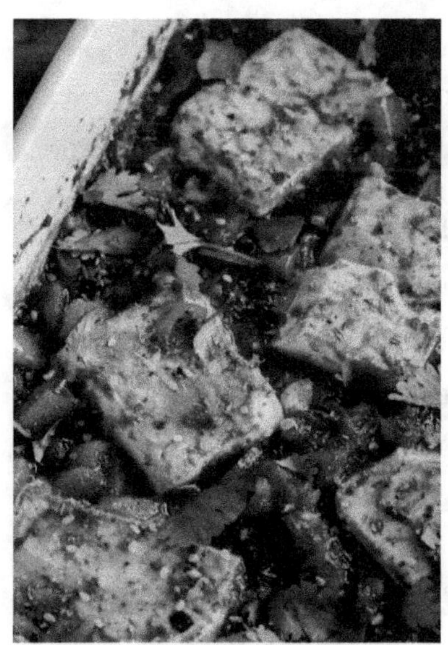

Tofu Shakshuka

Prep Time	Cook Time	Servings
10 min	30 min	4

INGREDIENTS:

- 1 tbsp olive oil
- 1 onion, sliced
- 2 garlic cloves, crushed
- 2 tbsp paprika
- 1 tsp cumin
- 2 x 14 oz cans chopped

tomatoes

- 1 red pepper, deseeded

and thinly sliced

- 2 tbsp parsley, finely

chopped

Method:

1. Preheat the oven to 400°F/Gas 6. Heat the olive oil in a flameproof casserole over medium heat. Sauté the onion for 5 minutes until soft; add the garlic and cook for another minute. Add the red pepper and sauté for another 5 minutes until tender. Stir in the paprika and cumin and cook for 1 minute. Stir in the chopped tomatoes and season with salt and pepper.

- 1 avocado, pitted and sliced

- Sea salt & freshly ground black pepper

- 3 ¼ cups pat-dried and diced firm tofu

Nutritional Value:

- Calories: 304
- Carbohydrates: 9 g
- Protein: 18.2 g
- Fat: 21.7 g

2. Place the diced tofu on top, cover with a lid, and let it simmer for 10 minutes. Remove the lid, transfer the casserole to the oven, and bake for 10 minutes until the tofu has crisped. Divide the dish between four plates and garnish with chopped parsley and avocado slices.

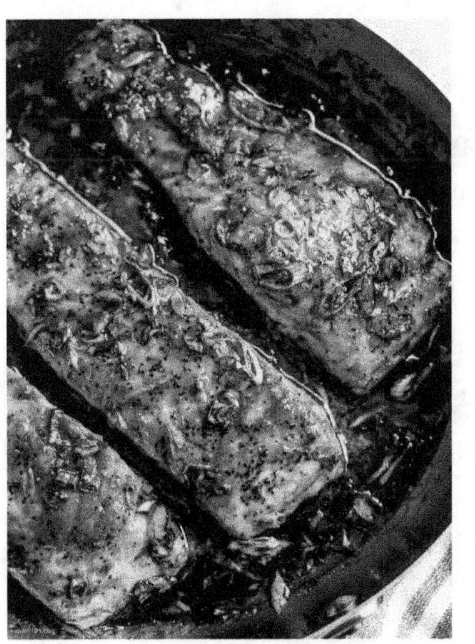

Salmon Teriyaki

Prep Time	Cook Time	Servings
5 min	15-20 min	4

INGREDIENTS:

- 4 tbsp tamari soy sauce

- 4 tsp grated ginger
- 4 x 5 oz salmon fillets
- 1 tbsp clear honey
- 2 tsp sesame oil
- 2 tbsp mirin

Method:

1. Preheat the oven to 425°F/Gas 7. Place the salmon fillets in a shallow baking dish.

2. Mix the clear honey, sesame oil, mirin, tamari soy sauce, and grated ginger in a bowl. Pour the mixture evenly over the salmon, ensuring that it is well-coated.

3. Bake the salmon for 15-20 minutes, or until it is cooked and easily flakes with a knife. Serve the salmon warm with steamed

tender-stem broccoli, asparagus, or bok choy as a side dish. It can also be enjoyed cold as part of a salad.

For serving:

- Steamed tender stem broccoli

- Asparagus
- Bok choy

Nutritional Value:

- Calories: 351
- Carbohydrates: 5.4 g
- Protein: 27.9 g
- Fat: 24.3 g

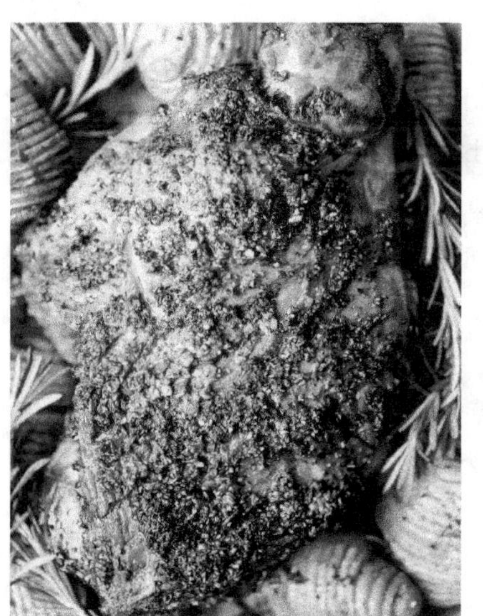

Roast Leg Of Lamb

Prep Time	Cook Time	Servings
5 min	15-20 min	4

INGREDIENTS:

- Olive oil
- 2 lb leg of lamb, bone-in
- 4 garlic cloves, sliced
- 2 sprigs rosemary,

leaves removed &

roughly chopped

- Sea salt and freshly

ground black pepper

Method:

1. Preheat the oven to 450°F/Gas 8.

2. Place the leg of the lamb in a roasting pan. Make ¾-in slits in the flesh and insert the sliced garlic and chopped rosemary into the slits. If the lamb has been refrigerated, allow it to come to room temperature.

3. Before cooking, drizzle the lamb with olive oil and season it with salt and pepper. Roast the lamb in the preheated oven for 15-20

For serving:

- Green beans

- Gratin potatoes

Nutritional Value:

- Calories: 481

- Carbohydrates: 0.9 g

- Protein: 42.8 g

- Fat: 34 g

minutes, then reduce the oven heat to 300°F/Gas 2 and continue roasting for an additional 20-25 minutes per 1 lb for medium-rare, or another 25-30 minutes per 1 lb for medium.

4. After cooking, allow the lamb to rest, covered with foil, for 10-15 minutes. Carve the lamb and serve it with green beans and gratin potatoes as desired.

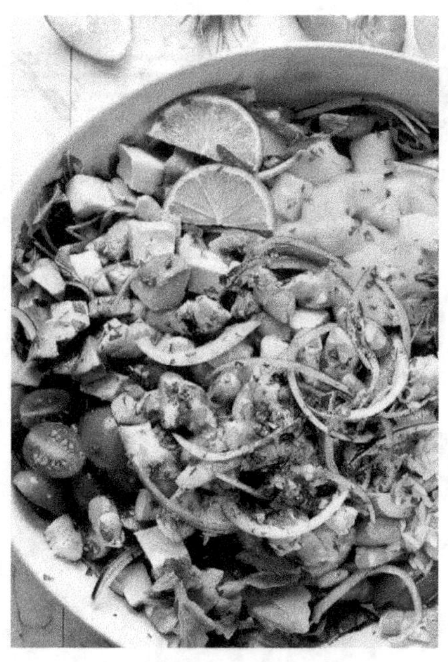

Prawn, Avocado, Grapefruit and Mango Salad

Prep Time	Cook Time	Servings
20 min	None	10

INGREDIENTS:

- Juice of 1 lime
- 1 diced mango
- 3 ¼ cups lamb's lettuce
- 2 avocados, pitted and

diced

- 4 ½ cups prawns,

cooked, peeled &

deveined

- 2 grapefruits, segments

separated & pith

removed

Method:

1. Place the diced avocado in a serving bowl and add the lime juice. Gently stir to coat the avocado and prevent browning. Add the prawns, grapefruit segments, diced mango, and lamb's lettuce to the bowl.

2. Combine the lemon juice, extra virgin olive oil, Dijon mustard,

262

For dressing:

- 4 tbsp lemon juice
- 1 tsp Dijon mustard
- 4 tbsp extra virgin

olive oil

- 2 tsp finely chopped

coriander

Nutritional Value:

- Calories: 225
- Carbohydrates: 11.7 g
- Protein: 13.6 g
- Fat: 13.7 g

and finely chopped coriander in a separate bowl to make the dressing. Stir well to combine.

3. Pour the dressing over the salad ingredients in the serving bowl and carefully toss to coat everything evenly. If desired, refrigerate the salad for 1 hour to allow the flavors to meld before serving.

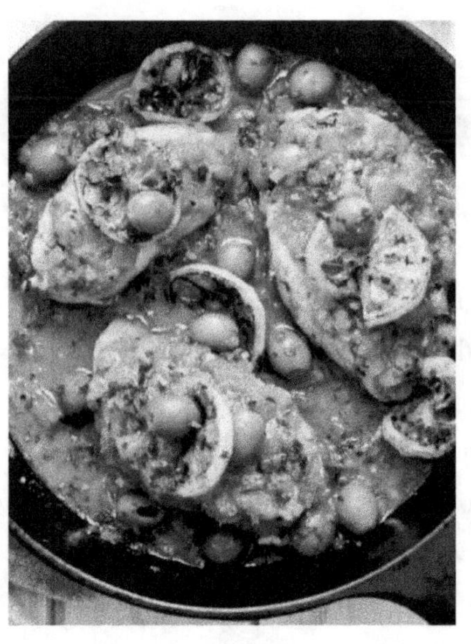

Chicken with Green Olives

Prep Time	Cook Time	Servings
5 min	1 hr	4

INGREDIENTS:

- 3 tbsp olive oil
- 4 chicken legs (thighs

and drumsticks)

- 1 onion, finely chopped
- 3 garlic cloves, sliced
- 1 tsp ground ginger
- 1 tsp ground turmeric
- 2 cups chicken bone

broth

- 1 tbsp coriander, chopped

Method:

1. In a flameproof casserole dish, heat the olive oil over medium heat. Brown the chicken legs in the oil, then remove and set them aside.

2. Add the chopped onion to the casserole dish and cook until translucent, approximately 5 minutes. Stir in the sliced garlic and spices (ground ginger and

ground turmeric), and cook for 3-5 minutes, not burning the spices.

3. Return the chicken legs to the casserole dish, then pour the chicken bone broth. Bring the mixture to a boil. Add the chopped coriander, chopped flat-leaf parsley, pitted green olives, lemon parts, and season with salt and pepper. Mix well to combine all the ingredients.

4. Reduce the heat to a simmer and cook for about 45 minutes or until the chicken is tender and easily separates from the bone.

4. Serve the chicken with basmati rice or quinoa

- 1 tbsp flat-leaf parsley, chopped

- 1 cup pitted green olives

- 1 lemon, cut into 8 parts

- Sea salt & freshly ground black pepper

For serving:

- Basmati rice

- Quinoa

Nutritional Value:

- Calories: 298
- Carbohydrates: 2.9 g
- Protein: 21 g
- Fat: 22.5 g

Beef and Liver Meatballs

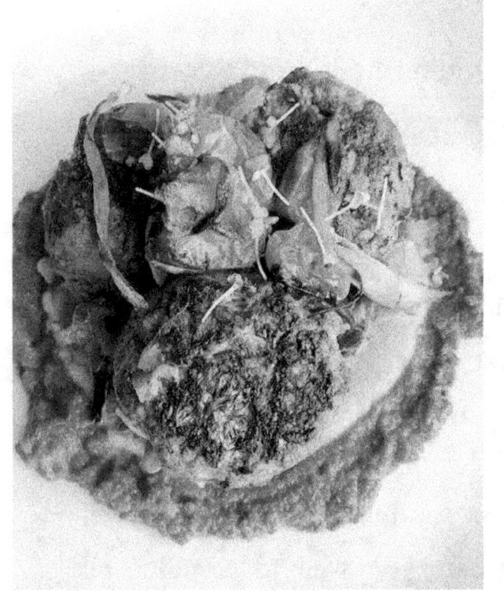

Prep Time	Cook Time	Servings
25 min	25-30 min	4

INGREDIENTS:

- 2 eggs
- ¼ tsp sea salt
- 1 lb minced beef
- 1 finely diced onion
- 3 tbsp grated Parmesan
- 1 cup finely diced
- chicken liver

Method:

1. Preheat the oven to 400°F/Gas 6 and line a tray with parchment paper.

2. Combine the chicken liver, minced beef, onion, sea salt, Parmesan, and eggs in a large bowl. Mix well using your hands until all the ingredients are thoroughly combined.

3. Wet your clean hands and shape the mixture into 12 balls, approximately 1 ¾ oz each. Place

- Wholegrain

or wild rice

- Tender stem

broccoli

Nutritional Value:

- Calories: 409
- Carbohydrates: 0.7 g
- Protein: 40.5 g
- Fat: 27 g

the meatballs on the prepared tray.

4. Bake in the preheated oven for 25-30 minutes or until the meatballs are cooked.

5. Serve the meatballs warm with wholegrain or wild rice and tender-stem broccoli.

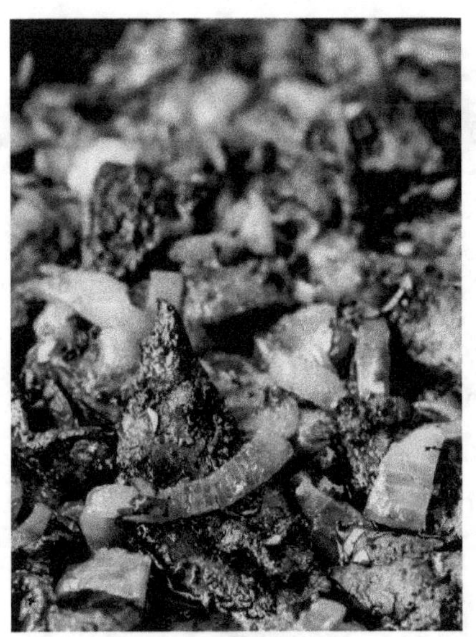

Liver, Onion and Sage

Prep Time	Cook Time	Servings
10 min	10 min	5

INGREDIENTS:

- 1 tsp sea salt
- 6 tbsp olive oil
- 1 onion, finely sliced
- 2 tbsp buckwheat flour
- 3 ¼ cups chicken liver, sliced into 3 strips
- 1 tbsp finely sliced sage leaves

Method:

1. Heat 1 tablespoon of olive oil over medium heat in a large frying pan. Add the onion and cook until translucent and tender, about 5 minutes. Remove from the pan and set aside.

2. In a bowl, combine the buckwheat flour and sea salt. Add the sliced chicken liver and toss until well-coated.

3. Heat the remaining olive oil in the pan over medium heat. Add the

For serving:

- Broccoli with

rice, quinoa, or

roasted sweet potatoes

Nutritional Value:

- Calories: 353

- Carbohydrates: 5.7 g

- Protein: 12.3 g

- Fat: 30 g

coated liver strips and cook for a few minutes, flipping them halfway through. The liver should still be slightly pink in the center.

4. Return the onions to the pan and add the sliced sage. Stir for a few more minutes.

5. Serve immediately with broccoli and your choice of rice, quinoa, or roasted sweet potatoes.

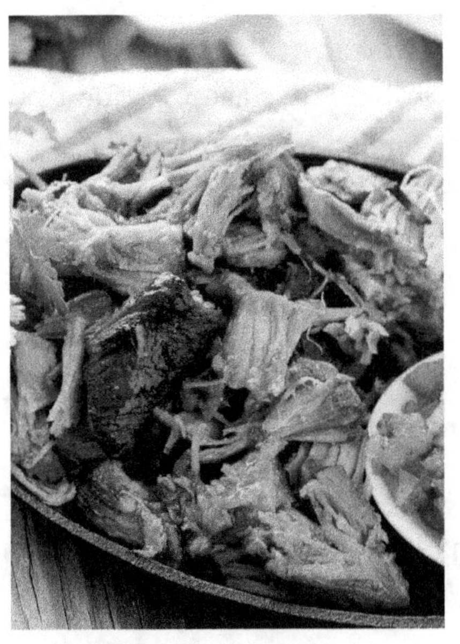

Pulled Pork

Prep Time	Cook Time	Servings
5 min	7-8 hr.	5

Method:

1. Preheat the oven to 475°F/Gas 9. Line a roasting tin with a large piece of foil.

2. Place the pork in the tin, fat side up.

3. Combine the smoked paprika, brown sugar, and salt in a small bowl. Rub the mixture over the pork.

4. Cook the pork in the preheated oven for about 40 minutes.

INGREDIENTS:

- 1 tbsp smoked

paprika

- 2 tbsp brown sugar
- 2 tbsp salt
- 2 lb boneless pork
- shoulder with fat

270

For serving:

- Cucumber, apple

- cider, and dill salad

- or red cabbage

Nutritional Value:

- Calories: 456

- Carbohydrates:

8.5 g

- Protein: 48.7 g

- Fat: 25.3 g

5. Reduce the heat to 300°F/Gas 2. Fold the foil around the pork, sealing it tightly. Continue cooking for 6-7 hours until the pork is tender and easily pulled apart with a fork.

6. Increase the heat back to 475°F/Gas 9 and cook the uncovered pork for another 10 minutes to crisp up the outer layer.

7. Remove the pork from the oven and let it rest for 30 minutes.

8. Shred the pork using two forks or pulling it apart with your hands.

9. Serve the pulled pork immediately with cucumber, apple cider, and dill salad or red cabbage.

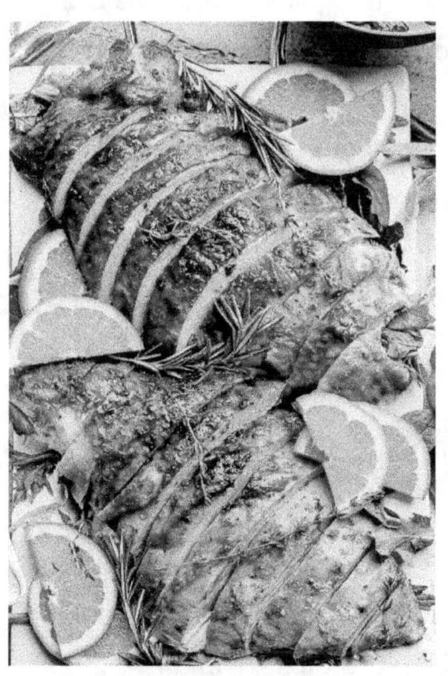

Orange and Herb-Roasted Turkey Breast Pork

Prep Time	Cook Time	Servings
10 min	40 min	4

INGREDIENTS:

- 1 1/3 lb turkey breast

- 2 tbsp olive oil
- 2 oranges, cut into 8 pieces

- Sea salt & freshly ground black pepper

- 2 tbsp sage, finely chopped

Method:

1. Preheat the oven to 425°F/Gas 7. Arrange the orange pieces in a roasting tin.

2. Season the turkey breast with salt and pepper, then place it on the oranges.

3. In a bowl, combine the olive oil and chopped herbs. Spoon the

272

- 2 tbsp rosemary, finely

chopped

- 2 tbsp thyme, finely

chopped

For serving:

- Rainbow salsa

Nutritional Value:

- Calories: 280

- Carbohydrates: 8.1 g

- Protein: 27.9 g

- Fat: 15 g

herb mixture evenly over the turkey.

4. Add 1 cup of water to the bottom of the roasting tin, ensuring it covers the oranges but not the bottom of the turkey.

5. Bake the turkey in the oven for 30-40 minutes or until the meat is cooked and the skin is brown and crisp. Monitor the water level during baking and add more to prevent the oranges from burning.

6. Discard the oranges and let the turkey breast rest for a few minutes at room temperature before slicing.

7. Serve the roasted turkey breast with rainbow salsa.

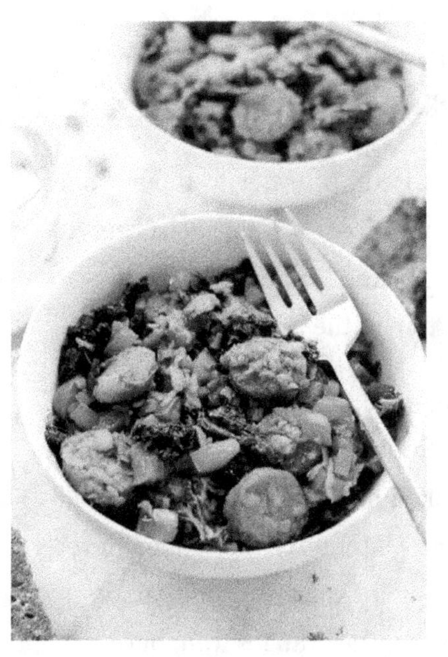

Sweet Potato, Kale and Sausage Bowl

Prep Time	Cook Time	Servings
20 min	45 min	4

INGREDIENTS:

- 4 tbsp olive oil
- 3 ¼ cups kale, stalks removed
- 2 apples, peeled, cored, & sliced
- 2 ½ cups sweet potato, peeled & diced

Method:

1. Preheat the oven to 400°F/Gas 6. Place the sweet potato on a baking tray, add half of the olive oil, season with salt and pepper, and stir to combine. Bake for 30 minutes or until the sweet potatoes are tender. Set aside.

2. Heat a frying pan over medium heat. Add the remaining olive oil and the sausage slices. Fry,

- Sea salt & freshly ground black pepper

- ¾ cup sausages, each cut into ½-in slices

For serving:

- Coriander or flat-leaf parsley

Nutritional Value:

- Calories: 368

- Carbohydrates: 37.2 g

- Protein: 7.1 g

- Fat: 21.2 g

stirring regularly, until the sausages are cooked through. Remove from the pan and set aside.

3. In the same pan, add the kale and stir for a few minutes until it is almost wilted.

4. Add the cooked sweet potatoes, sausages, and sliced apples to the pan. Stir for a few more minutes to allow the flavors to combine.

5. Serve the sweet potato, kale, and sausage mixture warm, garnished with coriander or parsley.

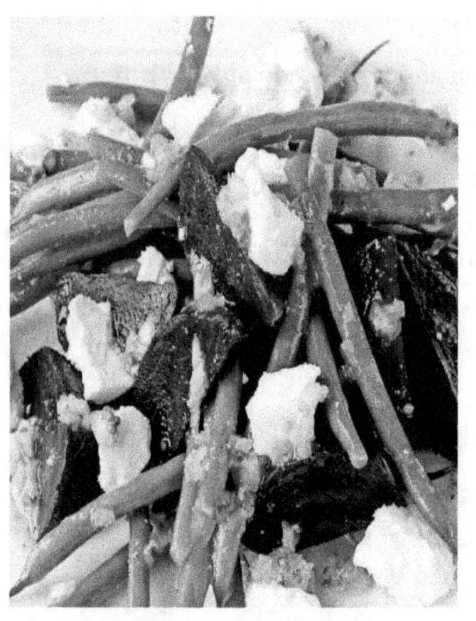

Beetroot and Goat's Cheese salad

Prep Time	Cook Time	Servings
20 min	None	4

INGREDIENTS:

For the dressing:

- 2 tbsp extra virgin olive oil
- 2 tbsp lemon juice
- 2 tsp Dijon mustard
- 3 ¼ cups watercress
- 8 eggs boiled, peeled, & halved

Method:

1. In a bowl, blend the dressing ingredients.

2. In a serving bowl, combine the watercress, diced beetroot, crumbled goat's cheese, chopped walnuts, and most of the parsley (saving some for garnish).

3. Pour the dressing over the salad ingredients and gently toss to

- 4 beetroot, cooked &

diced

- 1 ½ cups goat's cheese,

crumbled

- ½ cup walnuts, roughly

chopped

- 2 tbsp flat-leaf parsley,

chopped

Nutritional Value:

- Calories: 498
- Carbohydrates: 4.2 g
- Protein: 32.7 g
- Fat: 35 g

combine, being careful not to let the beetroot color the cheese.

4. Layer the halved boiled eggs on top of the salad.

5. Garnish with the remaining parsley.

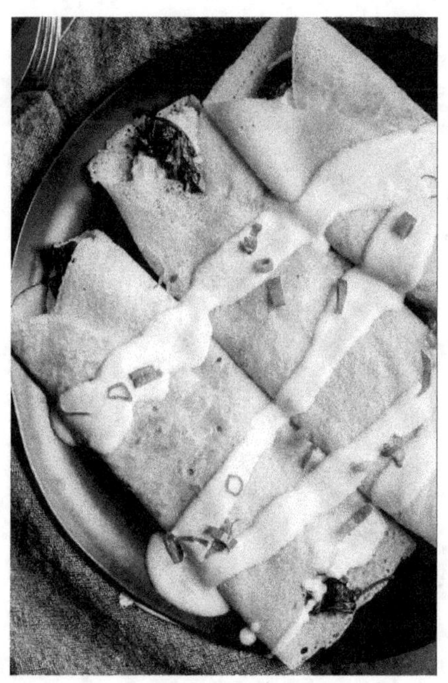

Chickpea Crêpe with Goat's Cheese and Asparagus

Prep Time	Cook Time	Servings
5 min	10 min	4

INGREDIENTS:

- 2 cups chickpea (gram) flour
- 2 tsp turmeric
- 1 tsp sea salt
- 2 tsp olive oil
- 3 oz goat's cheese

Method:

1. Combine 2 oz chickpea flour, 4 fl oz water, ½ teaspoon turmeric, and ¼ teaspoon salt in a blender. Blend until smooth.

2. Heat a frying pan over medium heat and add ½ teaspoon olive oil.

3. Pour the chickpea flour mixture into the pan, swirling it around to evenly cover the pan. Cook for 3-4 minutes, then flip the crêpe.

278

For serving:

- Steamed asparagus

- 2 avocados, pitted

& sliced

- 4 slices smoked

salmon

- Crème Fraiche

Nutritional Value:

- Calories: 269

- Carbohydrates: 25.6 g

- Protein: 12.7 g

- Fat: 12.9 g

4. Place a quarter of the goat's cheese on half of the crêpe and let it melt.

5. Fold it over the melted cheese once the crêpe is cooked on both sides.

6. Serve the crêpe with steamed asparagus, sliced avocado, smoked salmon, and crème fraiche on the side.

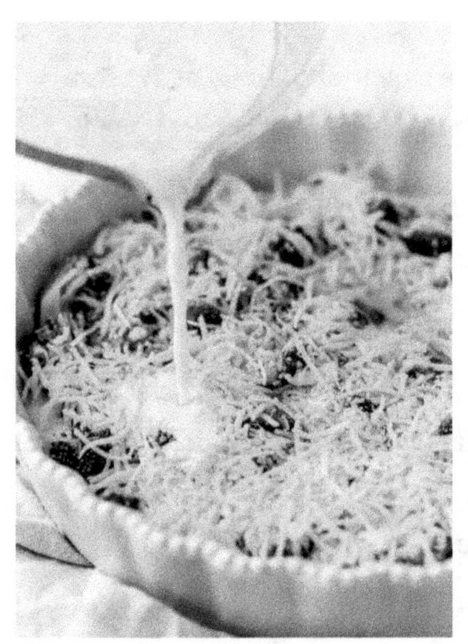

Crustless Broccoli Quiche

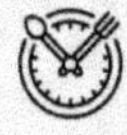

Prep Time	Cook Time	Servings
10 min	30 min	4

INGREDIENTS:

- 4 eggs
- 1 ½ cups crème fraiche
- 1 cup cheddar cheese, grated
- 1 ½ cups steamed broccoli, cut into small florets
- Sea salt and freshly ground black pepper

Method:

1. Preheat the oven to 400°F/Gas 6 and line a 9-in round oven tin with parchment paper.

2. Scatter the broccoli florets into the tin.

3. Whisk together the eggs, crème fraiche, and grated cheddar cheese in a large bowl. Season with salt and pepper.

280

For serving:

- Green side salad

Nutritional Value:

- Calories: 400
- Carbohydrates:

3.8 g

- Protein: 17.6 g
- Fat: 32.5 g

4. Pour the mixture over the broccoli in the tin, ensuring it is evenly distributed. Tap the tin gently on the tabletop to remove any air bubbles.

5. Bake in the oven for 30 minutes or until the quiche is set and golden.

6. Remove from the oven and let it cool slightly. Serve warm or cold with a green side salad.

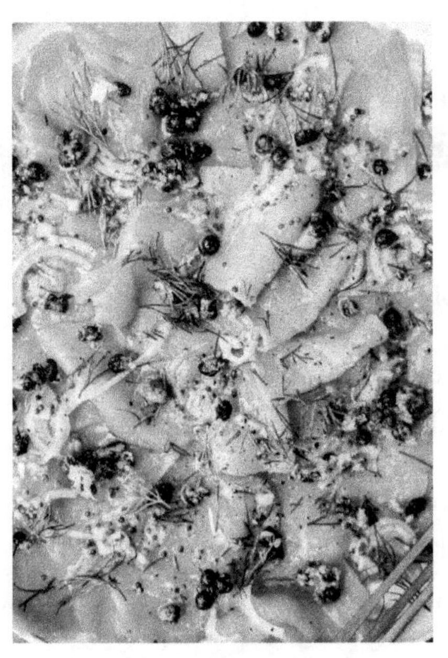

Tuna, Salmon and Mackerel Carpaccio

Prep Time	Cook Time	Servings
50 min	2 hr	5

INGREDIENTS:

- 10 oz tuna steak fillet
- 10 oz mackerel fillet
- 10 oz salmon fillet
- 3 ½ tbsp lime juice
- ½ cup lemon juice
- 3 ½ tbsp extra virgin

olive oil

- 3 tsp grated fresh ginger
- 2 ½ tbsp tamari soy sauce

Method:

1. Wrap each fish fillet individually in cling film and freeze for 24 hours. Remove from the freezer, discard the cling film, and let them sit at room temperature for a few minutes.

2. Using a sharp knife, carefully slice each fillet as thinly as possible. Place each fillet in a separate dish or arrange them together in one dish.

282

- ½ small fennel, finely

diced

- 1 tsp dill, finely

chopped

- ½ small red onion,

finely sliced

- 1 tbsp small capers

For serving:

- Wakame seaweed salad

- Rainbow salsa

Nutritional Value:

- Calories: 382

- Carbohydrates: 2.3 g

- Protein: 33.3 g

- Fat: 26.6 g

3. Drizzle the tuna with lime juice, the salmon with lemon juice, and the mackerel with olive oil. Refrigerate for 1 hour.

4. Mix the grated ginger and tamari soy sauce in a small bowl.

5. Just before serving, top the tuna with the ginger and tamari mixture, the mackerel with the diced fennel and chopped dill, and the salmon with the sliced red onion and capers.

6. Serve the carpaccio with a side of wakame seaweed salad and rainbow salsa.

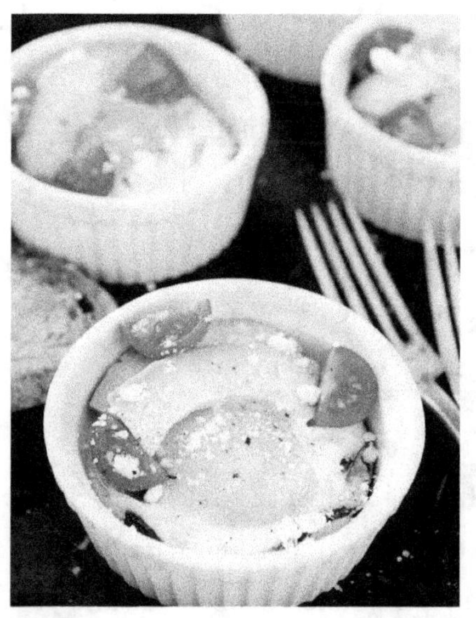

Baked Eggs with Spinach, Tomato & Feta

Prep Time	Cook Time	Servings
15 min	20 min	4

INGREDIENTS:

- 4 eggs
- 1 tsp paprika
- 1 ½ cups crumbled

feta cheese

- 2 cups passata
- 1 garlic clove, thinly

sliced

Method:

1. Preheat the oven to 200°C (425°F/Gas 7). Place the boiled potatoes at the bottom of an ovenproof dish.

2. Scatter the wilted spinach over the potatoes and pour the passata over it. Sprinkle half the sliced garlic on top and season with salt and pepper.

- 2 ¼ cups new potatoes,

boiled and cut into

chunks

- Sea salt and freshly

ground black pepper

- 2 ¼ cups baby

spinach, washed,

wilted,

& squeezed to remove

excess water

Nutritional Value:

- Calories: 316
- Carbohydrates: 20.2 g
- Protein: 19.9 g
- Fat: 17.2 g

3. Create four evenly spaced wells in the dish and carefully crack an egg into each well.

4. Sprinkle paprika and the remaining sliced garlic over the dish, then dot the crumbled feta cheese.

5. Bake for 15-20 minutes until the eggs are cooked to your liking.

6. Serve the baked eggs warm

28 Days Meal Plan

Day	Breakfast	Lunch	Snack/Dessert	Dinner
1	Rhubarb & Blueberry Smoothie	Brown Rice & Watercress Salad	Beetroot Crisps	Lamb Stew
2	Banana Shake	Sweet Potato Salad	Strawberry Soufflé Pancakes	Beef Spinach and Spices with Rice
3	Honey & Cinnamon Soy Milk	Oriental Rice Salad	Orange & Avocado Salad	Salmon Teriyaki

4	Fruit & Nut Shake	Roasted Dijon Chicken	Apple, Celery & Beetroot Salad	Mussels in white wine
5	Phyto Fruit Loaf	Baked Cod with Lemon Sauce	Rainbo w Salsa	Beef Bourguigno n
6	Scrambled Tofu	Corn Chowder with Garlic Prawns	Banana & Rice Pudding	Bacon, Mushrooms & Eggs Cauliflower Bowl
7	Banana Oat Crepes	Summer Salad	Tomato & Garlic Toast	Salmon Teriyaki
8	Sussex Soy Bread	Chicken Noodle Soup	Sardine & Avocado Wrap	Roast leg of lamb

9	Soy & Buckwheat crepes	Edamame Bean & Vegetable Soup	Phyto fix bars	Chicken with Green olives
10	Soy & Rice crepes	Mushroom & Mint Soup	Hummus (with rice cake)	Beef & Liver Meatballs
11	Crunchy Almond Granola	Carrot & Apricot Pate	Beetroot crisps	Tofu Shakshuka
12	Phyto Muesli	Tofu, Bean & Herb Stir-Fry	Cinnamon Apple Tart	Liver, Onion & Sage
13	Porridge with Spiced Fruit Compote	Baked Potatoes with spicy Soybeans	Coleslaw	Pulled Pork

14	Chili & Corn Fitter with Scrambled Eggs	Potato Skin with Broccoli & Tofu	Fruit Clafoutis	Orange And Herb-roasted Turkey Breast
15	Home-made Baked Beans	Bean Burgers	Parsnip & Apple Soup	Oven-Baked Eggplant Parmesan
16	Almond & Coconut Pancakes	Bean Tacos	Black Olive & Tuna Cake	Sweet Potato, Kale, & Sausage Bowl
17	Green Smoothie Bowl	Spanish omelet	Chewy Fruit Bars	Crust-less Broccoli Quiche

18	Berber Eggs	Salmon with Honey-Soy Glaze	Apple Walnut Coffee Rolls	Beetroot & Goat's Cheese salad
19	Phyto Sprinkles over Cereal	Nicoise Salad with Soy Dressing	Puy lentils, Ham & Feta Salad	Chickpea Crepe with Goat's Cheese Asparagus
20	Rhubarb & Blueberry Smoothie	Brown Rice & Watercress Salad	Three Bean Salad	Baked Eggs with Spinach, Tomato & Feta
21	Banana Shake	Sweet Potato Salad	Easy Egg Cups	Tuna, Salmon, & Mackerel Carpaccio

22	Honey & Cinnamon Soy Milk	Oriental Rice Salad	Phyto fix bars	Tofu Shakshuka
23	Fruit & Nut Shake	Roasted Dijon Chicken	Apple, Celery & Beetroot Salad	Mussels in white wine
24	Phyto Fruit Loaf	Baked Cod with Lemon Sauce	Rainbow Salsa	Beef Bourguignon
25	Scrambled Tofu	Corn Chowder with Garlic Prawns	Banana & Rice Pudding	Bacon, Mushrooms & Eggs Cauliflower Bowl
26	Banana Oat Crepes	Summer Salad	Tomato & Garlic Toast	Salmon Teriyaki

27	Sussex Soy Bread	Chicken Noodle Soup	Sardine & Avocado Wrap	Roast leg of lamb
28	Soy & Buckwheat crepes	Edamame Bean & Vegetable Soup	Phyto fix bars	Chicken with Green olives

Conclusion

Women searching for hormonal balance and relief from menopause symptoms through natural treatments will find The Menopausal Diet Book for older women to be a helpful resource. This comprehensive guide offers a lot of knowledge and helpful advice to assist women in navigating the difficulties of this stage of life with grace and vigor.

The Menopause Diet Book provides a comprehensive method to address these difficulties. Hormonal changes associated with menopause can result in a variety of physical and emotional changes. This book gives women the power to take charge of their physical and mental well-being throughout this transitional period by emphasizing dietary choices and applying natural therapies.

This book's focus on nutrition is one of its main advantages. Meal plans and dishes that have been carefully chosen are intended to enhance hormonal balance and lessen menopausal symptoms. The book teaches women how to customize their diets for hormone healing and general wellness by including certain foods and vitamins and minerals, such as estrogen-like substances and vital fatty acids.

The book also discusses a number of all-natural treatments that can help with menopausal symptoms. Readers can discover a variety of evidence-based methods to improve their well-being, from medicinal products to stress-relieving strategies. The necessity of consistent exercise, restful sleep, and stress reduction as key elements of an all-inclusive menopause support plan are also covered in the book.

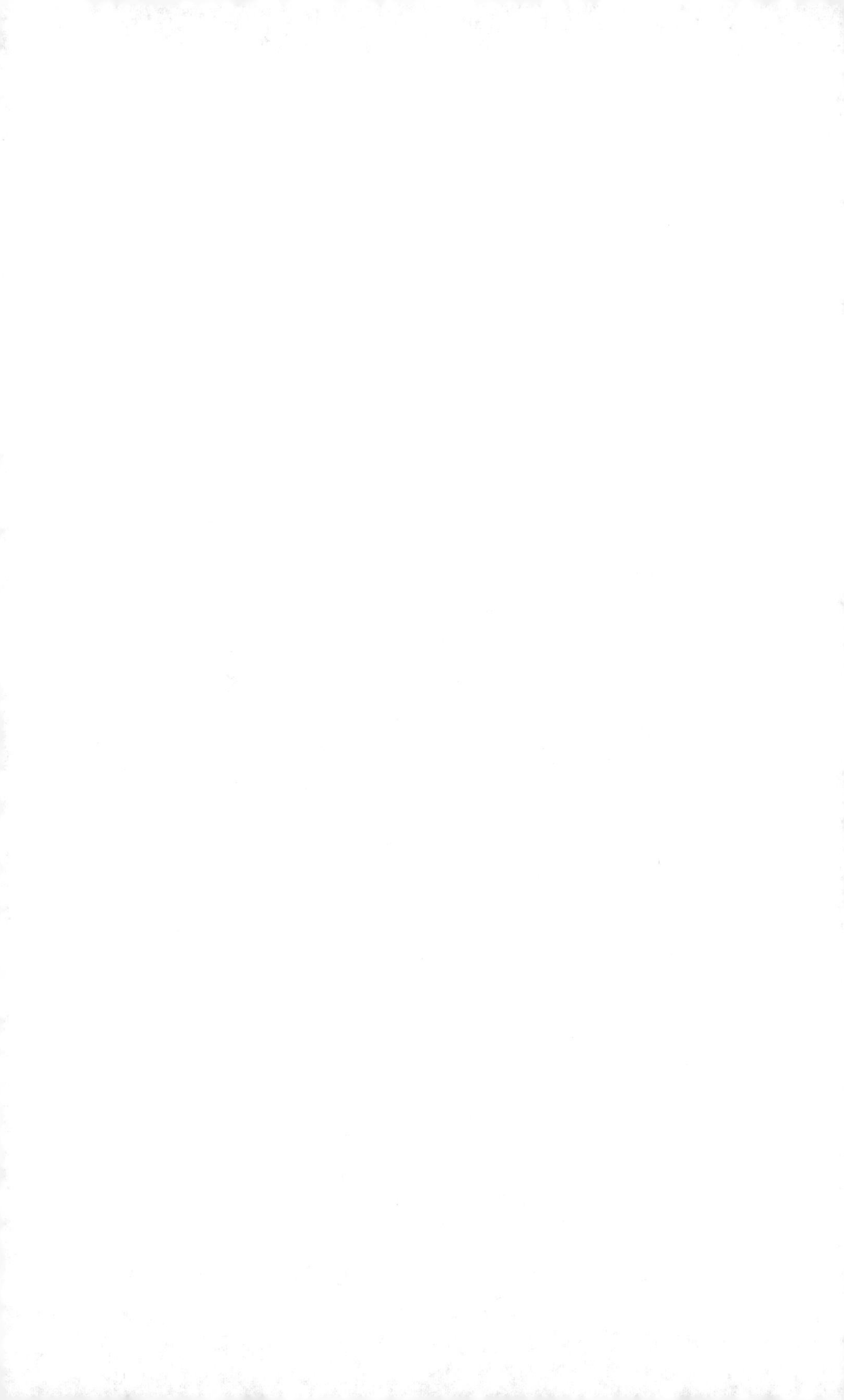

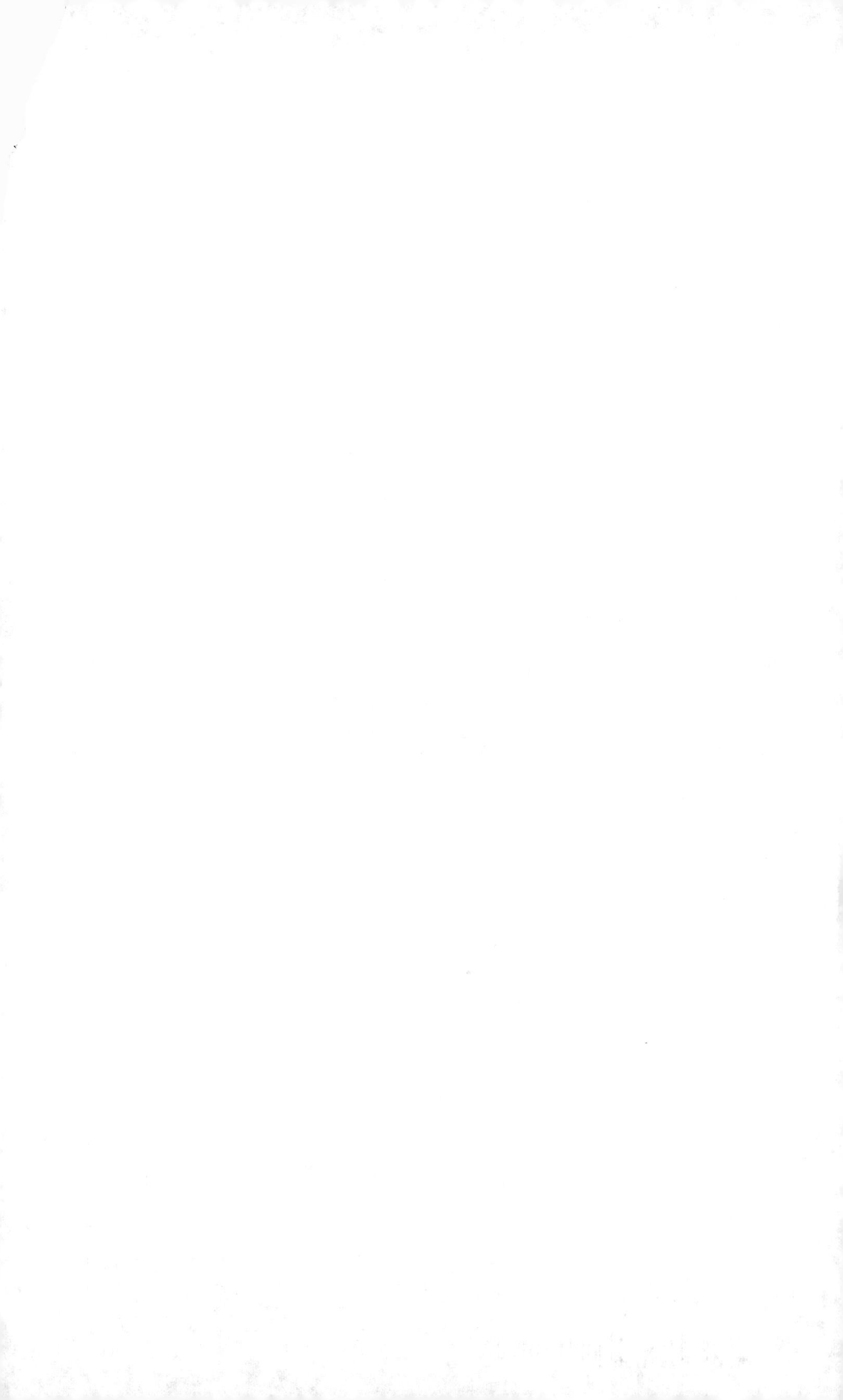